HATHA YOGA:
Developing the Body, Mind and Inner Self

by

Dee Ann Green Birkel, M.S.
Ball State University
Muncie, Indiana

eddie bowers publishing, inc
2600 Jackson Street
Dubuque IA 52001

ACKNOWLEDGEMENTS

I wish to thank many people for their contributions to this book. First, thanks to my husband, Lane for his support, editing and living with the project in his office while sharing his computer with me. Also thanks to my daughters Becky, Laura and Mary who have done yoga with me over the years. Also thanks to Becky for the Section on Acupuncture/ Acupressure and to my son, Jeff, daughter-in-law Tammy, and son-in-law Ronald who were all supportive and interested in the project.

A thank you to my photographer, Paul Troxell, for a job well done. And to the Ball State students from the yoga classes who offered to be models a big THANK YOU! - Maria Sharpe and Kevin Raidy who posed for the majority of the asanas; to Shawn Yancy who demonstrated yoga asanas while pregnant and to the athletes: Briseida Guzman, Mary Beth Singleton, Gena Rusch, Dave Keener, Roman Muller and Gary Telles. I will cherish your sharing and the memories of the photo sessions.

Thanks also to massage therapist, Ruth Ann Hobbs, to chiropractor, Dexter Nardella, and to Trager Practioner, Michael Sternfeld for sharing their knowledge and expertise with me. To my colleagues in the Womens Physical Education Department, the School of Physical Education and at Ball State University who have supported hatha yoga in the curriculum another big THANK YOU.

And to all of my yoga teachers and my yoga students who have all taught me so much. I wish to express my appreciation and gratitude.

And finally, thanks to Eddie, Carla and Sharon for bringing this book to the final stage that you are reading now.

NAMASTE.

Dee Ann
Fall, 1990.

eddie bowers publishing, inc.
2600 Jackson Street
Dubuque, Iowa 52001

ISBN 0-945483-07-4

Copyright © 1991, by *eddie bowers publishing, inc.*

TABLE OF CONTENTS

PREFACE

This book has grown from a need to have an appropriate manual for the college student. I have been teaching since 1977. There are many yoga books on the market, but I felt there is a need for a different type of book. This book is directed toward the beginning student with material that is easily understood and used in a practice session. Many of the ideas and content in this book are the results of a survey given to my students. They were asked to tell me what THEY wanted in a book and what THEY thought would be helpful to them.

Yoga is no longer regarded by our society as an activity that is mysterious. Thousands are learning and practicing yoga in their own living room via a videotape or a television program. Some become acquainted with yoga at a health/fitness spa and many have taken yoga at YMCA'S and YWCA'S, open universities, weekend workshops and on college campuses. Yoga has become an accepted form for helping with stress reduction as well as having a teaching format that is non-competitive and individualized.

Yoga has been recommended by physicians, psychologists, psychiatrists, chiropractors, massage therapists and athletic trainers to people of all sizes, shapes and ages. We have become more aware of our "whole self" and that we do not just consist of unrelated parts. We are interconnected and the learning of yoga assists in this discovery so that this marvelous machine, the human body and inner self, can reach its full potential.

The book will discuss the yoga exercises and how they help the body develop muscular strength, endurance, flexibility, balance, breath control and mental concentration. Let me stress that everyone is different and we come in all forms. Each of us is a unique individual and thus the approach to Hatha Yoga is one that encourages each person to work at a level that is comfortable.

This book includes check sheets as well as a list of references for supplemental reading. This book provides for college students in particular and any other beginning student of yoga a practical introductory guide to Hatha Yoga.

INTRODUCTION: What is Yoga?

When we treat Man as he is,
we make him worse than he is.
When we treat him as if he already were
what he potentially could be,
we make him what he should be."
Goethe (1749-1832)

I would like to define YOGA as a way of life that developed in India approximately 5,000 years ago. It is a system of working with the whole body. The word "YOGA" is derived from the Sanskrit word "yuj" (yoke), meaning to join or unite together all aspects of us as a person-our physical self, our mental self, our emotional self, our history, and our goals for the future. We are not just a body strengthening muscles, improving flexibility at the joints, reducing stress by relaxing, or improving energy and lung capacity by doing the breathing techniques. These are all important components but when they are all incorporated into one Hatha Yoga exercise session the effect on the body and the benefits gained are marvelous to experience. I have heard so many wonderful stories from my 4800-plus students since 1977 of how our class has helped them cope, improve some aspect of their life or even changed their lives in some way for the better. I would like to share with you the results of a research project conducted at Ball State University by Susan Gove Rudolph for her doctoral dissertation in 1981. The intent of the project was to determine if those 54 female students who participated in the ten week Hatha Yoga class could produce a change in self-concept. The results were compared with the 53 female students in an Effective Interpersonal Relationship Development class taught by Counselling Psychology and 53 in four randomly selected algebra classes. All of the subjects were given a questionnaire (Bills Index of Adjustment and Values) at the beginning and end of the ten week sessions. The students in the Hatha Yoga group indicated a significant change in self-concept ($p=.006$) but not the Counseling Psychology group ($p =.08$) or the comparison group of Algebra students ($p=.36$). As these young women participated in the Hatha Yoga class, the discrepancy between how they saw themselves and how they would like to be decreased. "The majority of the students who answered a Student Opinion Questionnaire felt that participation in the Hatha Yoga class had helped them become more aware of themselves, feel better about themselves and had helped them solve personal and/ or physical problems." (Rudolph, Abstract p. 4, See Resources) I was very excited about these findings as we now had proof of a scientific nature of the far reaching and positive effects of doing Hatha Yoga. Students at this stage in their life are very vulnerable and under pressure from society to be a certain way in regards to body build, looks, clothes, etc. and thus can feel dissatisfied with themselves quite easily. Through the participation in the yoga activity, (which was essentially the same that term as every other term before and since) we can conclude that young women can become more accepting of themselves, thus hopefully alleviating some unhappiness and stress in their life. This is an important contribution on the part of yoga to the overall lifestyle of an individual.

HATHA YOGA is one aspect of the multi-faceted nature of yoga. In the practice of Hatha Yoga the concentration is on the physical exercises, (the Asanas,) and the breathing techniques, (the Pranayama) and the learning of relaxation techniques. The word "Hatha" is really two words from Sanskrit -"HA" means Sun and "THA" means Moon. This implies that as the forces from the Sun and Moon interact upon us and keep us and our universe in balance, we are to strive for this balance in ourselves as well. The positive and negative forces can be unified as yoga is practiced.

YOGA IN THE UNITED STATES

The history of yoga is long and interesting. It is believed to have developed in Northern India about 5,000 years ago as a means of training soldiers. It wasn't until the 5th or 6th century B.C. that scholars say that an Indian philosopher, Pantanjali, formulated the early yoga teachings into a science of physical and mental health that are known today as the "Yoga Sutras." In 1841 Ralph Waldo Emerson, Henry David Thoreau and Bronson Alcott began an intellectual study of the Bhagavad Gita, in Concord, Massachusetts, where a small collection of Indian sacred books had been received. It was in 1893 that the first Indian teacher, Swami Vivekananda, came to the United States, arriving in Chicago to give a speech to the World Parliament of Religions. He stayed for two years giving lectures in Detroit, Boston, New York and Chicago. In 1899 he founded the New York Vedanta Society and four of his colleagues opened yoga centers (ashrams near Los Angeles and in San Francisco). The interest in yoga continued to grow with the arrival of more teachers from India: Paramahansa Yogananda in 1920; Swami Vishnudevanada, (1958) who started the Sivananda Yoga Centers, in Val Morin, Quebec, Montreal, New York City, and in Nassau in the Bahamas; Richard Hittlelman (1961) who started the first national television hatha yoga program; Swami Kriyananda who founded a residential community near Nevada City, California in 1968; Swami Satchidananda (1966) who became known as the "Guru of Woodstock"; the students of Sri Krishnamacharya who made a tremendous impact on the American Hatha yoga scene and who are still active - the first woman teacher Indra Devi (1947), B.K.S. Iyengar (1973) Pattabhi Jois (1975), T.K.V. Desikachar (son of Krishnamacharya, 1976). Lilias Folan (1970) launched the first PBS-TV series "Lilias, Yoga & You, which was carried by over 200 stations in 1977. Swami Rama of the Himalayan Institute (1970) was involved in the research conducted at the prestigious Menninger Foundation in Topeka, Kansas where he demonstrated the "yogic control over involuntary autonomic nervous system function, including heartbeat, pulse rate and skin temperature", which led to the development and growth of the science of biofeedback. Yoga has thus become assimilated into our American culture and is not now being presented in a rigid, religious style but more as a philosophy or a way of life.

INTERNATIONAL YOGA SCENE

Yoga, like music, art, and sports, transcends the globe. One of the most exciting aspects of learning yoga is that no matter where you are in the world you will probably be able to find a class or a friend who also practices yoga. There are many yoga centers throughout the 'Western World' of Europe, England, North and South America as well as in the desirable resort areas of the islands in the Mediterranean, Pacific, Gulf of Mexico and the Atlantic ocean. Many of the leading teachers of one country will travel and do workshops around the world. The masters of yoga from India are well known among the yoga teachers of the world.

It is possible to refer to the summer issue of the *Yoga Journal* for a directory of yoga retreats, camps, trips, teacher training centers and teachers throughout the world. (refer to Resource.)

POTENTIAL FOR SELF GROWTH

The benefits gained from doing yoga are many and varied depending on the individual's needs. But in general it is safe to say that the basic flexibility, muscular strength, and endurance of the person doing yoga will be enhanced. Also the awareness of the breath and how the body can control and use the breath for raising energy levels and to calm the self is discovered. One of yoga's main contributions toward self growth is the awareness of the value of relaxation and ways to still the body and the mind. Many students develop a greater awareness of the marvelous ways in which the body is interconnected and how the mind can work with the physical self in a more harmonious manner. There are techniques in how yoga is done that can be transferred to other exercise practices as well.

SUMMARY

Yoga is like any activity you undertake- you get out of it what you put in. What you bring to it in the way of interest and awareness will enhance what you then will see as benefits. Read on now for some basic suggestions on how best to develop and continue your interest in hatha yoga.

RESOURCES

Books
Boyd, Doug. *Rolling Thunder*. New York, N.Y.: Dell Publishing Co. Inc. 1974.
Carr, Rachael. *Be a Frog, A Bird or A Tree*. Garden City, N.Y.: Doubleday and Co. Inc. 1973.
Kiss, Micchaeline. *Yoga for Young People*. Indianapolis, IN.: Bobbs Merrill Co. Inc. 1971.
Lidell, Lucy. *The Sivananda Companion to Yoga*. New York, N.Y.: Simon & Schuster. 1983.
Winding, Eleanor. *Yoga for Musicians and Other Special People*. Sherman Oaks, CA.: Alfred Publishing Co., Inc. 1982.

Publications
American Health Fitness of Body and Mind, 28 West 23rd Street, New York, N.Y. 10010.
New Realaties; Oneness of Self, Mind and Body. 4000 Albemarle St., NW, Washington, DC 20016.
New Age Journal, P. O. Box 53275, Boulder, CO 80321-3275.
Yoga Journal, 2054 University Ave. Berkely, Ca 94794-9975.

Articles
Kunes, Ellen. "No Sweat Fitnes," *Working Woman*, April 1990. p.119,20.

Dissertations
Collins, Lorrie Ann. *Stress Management and Yoga*. Doctoral Thesis, Indiana University, 1982.
Rudolph, Susan Gove. *The Effect on the Self Concept of Participation in Effective Interpersonal Relationships Development Classes*. Doctoral Thesis, Ball State University, Muncie, IN. 1981.

Organizations
Iyengar Yoga Institute of San Francisco. 2404 27th Avenue, San Francisco, CA 94116.
Sivanada Ashram Yoga Retreat, Box N7550, Paradise Island, Nassau, Bahamas (809)326-2402.

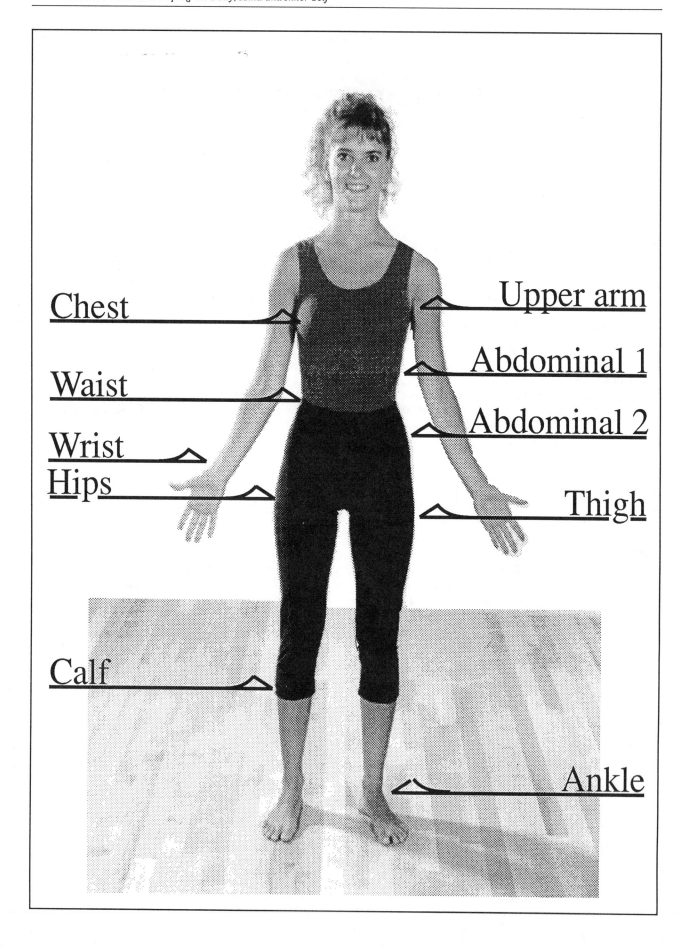

Chest

Waist

Wrist

Hips

Calf

Upper arm

Abdominal 1

Abdominal 2

Thigh

Ankle

YOGA BASICS

Don't believe what your eyes are telling
All they show is limitation.
Look with your understanding,
find out what you already know..."
Richard Bach, *Jonathan Livingston Seagull*

SELF ASSESSMENT

To be able to attain as much as possible from your involvement with hatha yoga it is helpful to take a reflective look at your self - your whole self. Who are YOU? What are your hopes and aspirations? What is your lifestyle like in regard to healthful living? Do you drink, eat, work, or smoke to excess? What are your eating habits? How do you handle stress? Do you exercise now, in the past, or have plans for the present and the future? Do you have any chronic health concerns such as epilepsy, diabetes, migraine headaches, old injuries, pre-menstrual tension etc.? How do you manage your time? Are your relationships with parents, siblings, room-mates, friends, special friends what you want them to be? What are your strengths? What do you LIKE about yourself?

Take a few moments now and write a letter to yourself discussing what ever you think would benefit YOU. You can use the above suggestions but feel free to expand and include anything you want. Now that you have communicated to the very important YOU, why not set a few goals for yourself based upon what developed in your letter? Be realistic - and don't set too many or ones that are unattainable at this point in your life. Later, in a few weeks, reread your letter and at the end of this term or 15 weeks write yourself another letter relating to the content of your first one. Are there changes in you and how you see who YOU are now? Ask yourself the question — Did yoga have a part in this? The purpose of this exercise is to help you become more aware of your whole self and your potential.

It is also helpful to complete the Stress Releases and Safety Valves, (Table 2.1 on page 8) now and refer to Unit 5 for more information if your score indicates that you are prone to stress problems. Also there is a Health History Questionnaire (Table 2.2 on page 9) which will bring to your attention some other aspects of you and your life and your future.

BODY COMPOSITION AND FLEXIBILITY

It is also meaningful to assess your physical self. This can be done by following the directions for doing the height, weight, girth measurements and the flexibility tests and recording them on Body Analysis Record Form (Table 2.3). You will see that there are three columns for recording your data - Now, after 7 weeks of yoga and again at the end of 15 weeks of yoga. Doing it in this manner will allow you to see changes that are developing.

Weight

Do in your bare or stocking feet, and light weight clothes or in your underwear if possible. Record to nearest 1/4 pound.

Height

Do in your bare or stocking feet, stand erect and have a friend record your height to the nearest 1/4 inch.

Girth Measurements

Referring to the sketch of the body (Fig. 2.1) for the location of each site to be measured follow these directions and record your circum-ference to the nearest 1/2 inch. Please keep the tape level. Measure your right arm and the right leg and overlap the tape to get an accurate reading.

Chest: Place the tape over the nipples of the chest and have a friend read the tape in the middle of the back, this allows you to adjust the tape to keep it level.

Abdominal 1: Place the tape just over the bottom of the rib cage.

Waist: Place the tape at the narrowest site for women and for men where you wear your belt.

Abdominal 2: Place the tape over the top of the hip bone (iliac crest on the pelvis).

Hips: Place the tape low over the pubic bone.

Thigh: Near the crotch and keep the tape level!

Calf: Place the tape over the fullest part- where the leg curves.

Ankle: Place the tape just above the bone.

Upper arm: Place the tape near the armpit and keep level!

Wrist: Place the tape just below the bone - toward the hand.

In (Table 2.4) you can refer to some Recommended Girth Measurements for Men and Women. These are just a reference if you should want one. No one is expected to be exactly as this would suggest (see page 8).

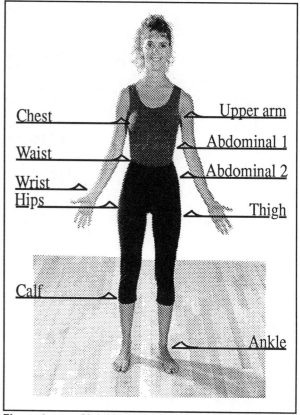

Figure 2.1. *Girth Measurements*

Resting Pulse

Sit quietly for ten minutes. Find your pulse in your neck or on your wrist and count for 30 seconds and then multiply the number by two giving your self a pulse count for 1 minute. A pulse in the range of the sixties or low seventies is considered to be normal. The lower the pulse the less your heart is working at rest. If you have had caffeine or are under stress your pulse could be elevated. A good time to take the pulse for a more accurate count is in the morning just before you get out of bed. As you further your yoga practice and develop your ability to relax, the resting pulse should lower.

Table 2.4.	**Recommended Girth Measurements**	
Area	**Women**	**Men**
Chest	same as hips	same as hips
Abdominal 1		
Waist	10" less than chest	5-7" less than chest
Abdominal 2		
Hips	same as chest	same as chest
Thigh	6" less than waist	8-10 " less than waist
Calf	6-7" less than thigh	7-8" less than thigh
Ankle	5-6" less than calf	6-7" less than calf
Upper arm	twice the size of wrist	twice the size of wrist

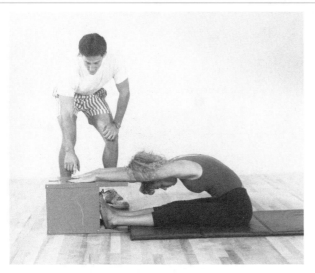

Figure 2.2. *Sit and Reach*

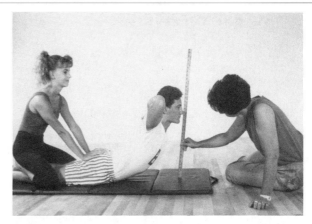

Figure 2.3. *Trunk Lift*

Flexibility

Sit and Reach

This test will measure the flexibility of your back and your hamstring muscles on the back of the thigh. To check your flexibility in these areas you will need a "flex - box " (Fig. 2.2) or a chair, a footstool, or a bench laid on its side, as well as a yardstick or meter stick placed on the edge of the chair with the number 10 on the yardstick (or 25.5 on the meter stick) lined up with the edge of the chair seat. Please follow the instructions.

1. Do a few stretching exercises to gently warm up the muscle groups of the back and legs (See Unit 3 preparation poses).
2. Remove shoes and wear loose clothing.
3. Sit on the floor placing the soles of your feet against the chair seat, and keeping your legs straight.
4. Place fingertips on your shoulders, IN-HALE, and reach toward the ceiling, straightening arms, lifting ribs, and contracting the abdominal muscles. Then EXHALE and lean forward as far as you can comfortably reach WITHOUT bending your knees. Read the number on the measuring stick where your fingertips touched. If it is beyond the number 10, subtract 10 from the number and write down + _____. If you touched a number from 1 to 10, subtract your number from 10 and write down -_____.

Trunk Lift

This flexibility test is similar to a yoga pose that you will be learning. If you have injured your back please don't do it now. If you chose to do it please follow the instructions.

1. Using three partners, one person lies on their abdomen with the fingers inter-locked and hands behind the neck, one partner is straddling the legs and places the hands with the fingers pointing toward the floor on the buttocks and the tops of their feet on the partners ankles to hold the legs down. The third partner is by the head of the person doing the lift (see Fig. 2.3).
2. The partner on the bottom will inhale and LIFT their trunk upward. The third partner will place a measuring stick in front of their chin and will quickly record the number of inches (or centimeters) the chin is from the floor.
3. The partner doing the lift will exhale and LOWER down with control

Hints: Do NOT jerk up quickly and force the body. This should be a gentle lift using the breath and done with control.
Do NOT do this test if you have ever injured the lumbar back or have a problem with the sciatiac nerve.

Table 2.1.   *Stress Releases and Safety Valves*

I do well	I'm average	Need to improve	
5	3	1	*(Place a check in the appropriate column. Try to be completely honest.)*
____	____	____	1. "Owning" my own stress (not blaming others).
____	____	____	2. Knowing my level of optimum stress (the level of stress that allows you to do your best without becoming destructive).
____	____	____	3. Balancing work and play (scheduling time for play).
____	____	____	4. Loafing more (learning to do nothing at times and feel okay about it).
____	____	____	5. Getting enough sleep and rest rather than ending up with what is left over at the end of the day (scheduling adequate sleep).
____	____	____	6. Refusing to take on more than I can handle (learning to say no).
____	____	____	7. Working off tension (hard physical effort on a regular basis).
____	____	____	8. Setting realistic goals (goals that can be achieved within a reasonable time frame).
____	____	____	9. Practicing relaxation (meditating with music or biofeedback).
____	____	____	10. Slowing down (taking pleasure in every moment rather than rushing through life).
____	____	____	11. Putting emphasis on being rather that doing (being a person others like to be around is more important than "doing" many activities).
____	____	____	12. Managing my time, including planning for time alone (setting priorities and doing those things that are most important).
____	____	____	13. Planning regular recreation (recreation is a complete change of pace and something that is fun to do).
____	____	____	14. Having a physical fitness program (having a specific plan for strenuous exercise).
____	____	____	15. Avoiding too much caffeine (limiting coffee and cola drinks).
____	____	____	16. Emphasis good nutrition in diet (learning about nutrition and avoiding junk foods).
____	____	____	17. Avoiding alcohol or other chemicals to deal with pressure (dependency on alcohol or drugs deals with symptoms rather than the problem).
____	____	____	18. Avoiding emotional "overload" (taking on problems of others when you are under stress is destructive).
____	____	____	19. Selecting emotional "investments" more carefully (of things we can get involved with that call for emotional involvement, it is necessary to choose carefully).
____	____	____	20. Giving and accepting positive "strokes" (being able to express positive things to others and receive positive comments in return is an achievement).
____	____	____	21. Talking out troubles and getting professional help if needed (being willing to seek help is a sign of strength rather than weakness).

Score Yourself

If you scored between 21 and 50, there are several areas you need to develop to better release your stress. It might be a good idea to discuss some of your answers with a counselor or close friend.

If you scored between 51 and 75, you have discovered a variety of ways to deal effectively with stress. Make a note of those items you checked "need to improve" and work on strategies to help you move to the "I'm Average" box.

If your score was 75 or greater - congratulations. You apparently have found some excellent ways to deal with frustration and the complexities of life. Stay alert to protect the valuable skills you have acquired.

Mental Fitness: A Guide to Emotional Health, Merrill F. Raber, M.S.W., Ph.D., and George Dyck, M.D., pages 23 and 24.

Table 2.2.   *Health History Questionnaire*

Name_____ Age_____ Student I.D.#_____

Date of Last Medical Check-up_____ Telephone_____ Date_____

Hour Class Meets_____ Year in School _____ Major_____

Please identify conditions that pertain to you.

_____	Heart problems	_____	Sleep disorders
_____	Blood Pressure	_____	Smoking
_____	Chest pain and discomfort	_____	Drinking excessively
_____	Family history of heart disease	_____	Eating disorders
_____	Allergies	_____	Scoliosis
_____	Asthma *Injuries to:*	_____	Cervical (Neck)
_____	Diabetes	_____	Thoracic (Upper back)
_____	Epilepsy	_____	Lumbar (Lower back)
_____	Severe headaches-fainting	_____	Knees
_____	Hernia	_____	Ankles
_____	Menstrual problems	_____	Foot
_____	Pregnant	_____	Shoulder

Please list any other conditions that you think are important to bring to the attention of your instructor.

_____

_____

Please list any medications that you take regularly. _____

_____

Letter to Me

Date_____

Dear Me _____

Table 2.3.   *Body Analysis Record Form*

Name _____   Class _____   Sec._____

	Start	**Middle**	**15th Week**
Date	_____	_____	_____
Weight	_____	_____	_____
Height	_____	_____	_____

Girth Measurements: *Standing - tape level, and refer to Unit 2 for complete instructions.*

Chest-fullest	_____	_____	_____
Abdominal 1 - over ribs	_____	_____	_____
Waist-narrowest	_____	_____	_____
Abdominal 2 - over stomach	_____	_____	_____
Hips- over pubic bone	_____	_____	_____
Right Thigh- near crotch	_____	_____	_____
Right Calf- fullest	_____	_____	_____
Right Ankle- above bone	_____	_____	_____
Right Upper arm- near armpit	_____	_____	_____
Right Wrist- below the bone	_____	_____	_____
Resting Pulse	_____	_____	_____

Flexibility

Sit and Reach (record + or - number)	_____	_____	_____
Trunk Lift	_____	_____	_____

HATHA YOGA PRACTICE GUIDELINES

Please read now the following suggestions for participating in a safe and fun hatha yoga session. Most of these recommendations apply to all forms of exercising and are good exercise habits to establish.

1. Do the yoga poses 1 1/2 to 2 hours following eating.
2. Empty the bladder and bowels.
3. Don't chew gum.
4. Don't wear large earrings or a lot of jewelry.
5. Clothing should be comfortable and allow for movement - NO JEANS! Sweat shirts and pants are too warm and don't allow you to monitor your alignment in the yoga poses.
6. Be in bare feet so that you have better contact and feedback regarding balance.
7. Practice in a well ventilated room and avoid being in a draft.
8. Breathe through the nose with the mouth closed. INHALE on the expanding movements and EXHALE on contracting movements. Breathe normally during the static stretching phase.
9. Do 3-4 repetitions of each asana.
10. If possible check your asanas in a mirror to correct your alignment
11. Don't strain- go to the "edge" of your stretch and back off slightly.
12. Concentrate on how your body is feeling and reacting to the activity-involve your mind so that you are more aware of your progress.
13. Practice in the early morning is fine but the body is a little stiffer then so be patient and warm up with gentle stretches.
14. Evening practice is good as it helps remove the tension of the day and refreshes the mind and body.
15. Always end your practice time with relaxation- you deserve it.

You are
> *never given a wish*
> *without also being given*
> *the power to make it true.*

You may
> *have to work for it*
> *however.*
...Richard Bach, *Illusions*

SUMMARY

Now that you found out some very important information about your self you are ready to begin learning the yoga poses and how they can benefit you. Unit 3 will present to you this information so read on.

RESOURCES

Publications
Ingber, D. "Yoga, the Impossible Science", *Science Digest,* February, 1982. p. 28-9.

SUN SALUTE

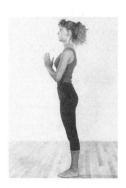

A. Beginning Pose: Exhale. (see figure 3.12 on page 18)

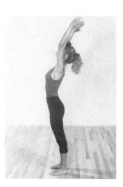

B. Slight Arch: Inhale. Tighten buttocks, lift rib cage and don't dorp head back.

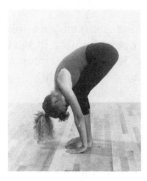

C. Standing Forward Bend. Exhale. Place hands beside feet.

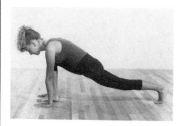

D. Lunge: Inhale. Take Right foot back. (see figure 3.29 on page 34)

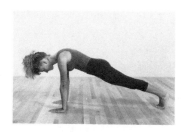

E. Plank: Hold the breath. (see figure 3.30 on page 34)

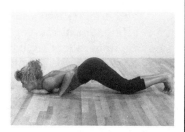

F. Knees & Chest: Exhale. Lower the knees to mat, chest between hands.

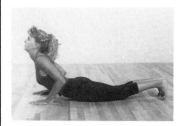

G. Cobra: Inhale. (see figure 3.13 on page 19)

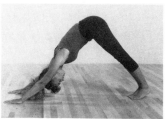

H. Dog: Exhale. (see figure 3.21 on page 25)

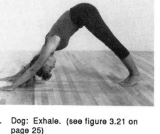

I. Lunge: Inhale. Bring Right foot up between hands. (see figure 3.29 on page 34)

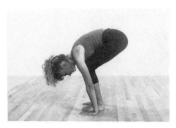

J   Standing Forward Bend: Exhale. Bring Left leg up.

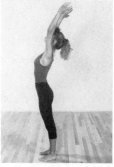

K. Slight Arch: Inhale. Tighten buttocks and lift rib cage.

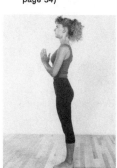

L. NAMASTE: Exhale. Hands together.

Repeat the routine again reversing the feet in the Lunge.

ASANAS: Hatha Yoga Poses

*"I hear and I forget
I see and I remember
I DO and I understand"*
A Chinese Proverb

BREATH

This chapter will introduce you to the yoga poses or "asanas." These exercises are gentle to your body if YOU do them gently. Always move into the pose with control and hold the static stretch or position for approximately ten seconds, and then with control, return to your starting position. A basic concept when doing yoga is to use your breath which gives you energy and contributes to your control. Inhale when the body is opening or expanding and exhale when you contract. Keeping your breath connected to the physical movement helps keep the oxygen intake up so the muscles will be comfortable with the exercise task you are asking them to perform.

COUNTERPOSE

Another concept that is a part of doing yoga, along with coordination of the breath to the exercise, is to use a "counter pose" to balance the body. For example, if you have done a pose that contracts the muscles of the back, then you follow with a pose that will gently stretch that muscle group. This can apply to all areas of the body. Muscle imbalance can be the cause of postural aches and pains. Hatha yoga helps bring this problem to your attention and will help you become aware of habits regarding your sitting, standing and walking practices which you may want to improve. You are encouraged to refer to Appendix B on page 108, a chart of the muscles, to familiarize yourself with the names as they will be used in the directions and discussions of the yoga asanas.

CONCENTRATION

A third concept that is an integral part of yoga practice is "concentration"- have your mind FEELING what the physical body is experiencing; feeling the energy needed to do the asana and then feeling the relaxation flow through you when you release the contraction or come out of the position. This feedback can only happen when you have your mind involved and go inward to monitor your self.

Everytime that you do the asanas you will want to incorporate the concepts described 1) coordinate the breath to the asana, 2) concentrate on what is being felt- the energy and the relaxation and 3) do a counter pose.

PREPARATION POSES

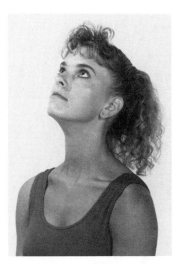

Figure 3.1. *Neck stretch*

Neck Stretch

Benefits: Improves the range of motion in the neck.
Precautions: Go very slowly if you have problems in the cervical vertebrae. Do not FORCE.
Directions: Sitting with back erect gently bring the chin to the chest and lift the head up to gaze at ceiling. Do NOT drop head back.
Breath: Inhale as lower and exhale as raise.

Neck Turn

Benefits: Improves the range of motion in the neck.
Precautions: Go very slowly if you have problems in the cervical vertebrae. Do Not FORCE;
Directions: Sitting with back erect gently turn the head from side to side noticing that it is kept level and how far you are able to comfortably turn before feeling resistance. Notice also a possible difference from the right and left side.
Breath: Inhale as you turn to side and exhale as you return to the center.

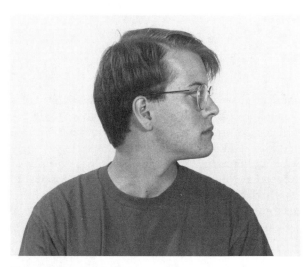

Figure 3.2. *Neck turn*

Body Rolls

Benefits: Gently stretches the back, shoulders and legs.
Precautions: If you have injured your neck do not roll back too far. Do gently on a padded surface. This could aggravate an injury to the tailbone.
Directions:
1. Sitting with knees bent and hands holding the back of the thighs, roll back up onto your shoulders and then rock back up. Repeat.
2. With knees bent, set your heels on mat and reach between your legs to hold your toes. Fold your Right leg in toward the body and then the Left leg and lean forward, Rock back as before and unfold your legs gently stretching them. Fold the legs back in and rock up and repeat folding the Left leg in first. Laugh if you want! Classes always do.
Breath: Inhale and exhale as roll back, inhale as rock forward.

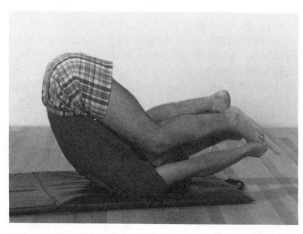

Figure 3.3. *Body rolls*

Knee Thigh Stretch (Bhadrasana)

Benefits: Improves the flexibility of the hip and knee.

Precautions: Be careful if you have injured your knees.

Directions: Sit with back erect and soles of feet together, hands placed on thighs. Gently press down until you feel a gentle stretching and then hold for 10 seconds. Repeat. Notice where your legs are in relation to the mat and notice how tight or flexible you feel.

Breath: Breath normally.

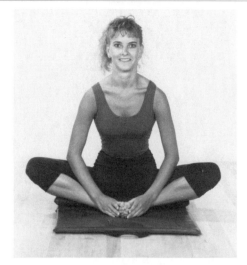

Figure 3.4. *Knee thigh stretch*

One Knee to Chest

Benefits: Improves the flexibility of the back, knee and hip. Also known as the gas reliever pose.

Precautions: Place hand on the thigh behind the lower leg and knee.

Directions: Lie on the back, bending the Right knee and draw the bent leg toward the chest. Change to the Left leg and repeat.

Breath: Inhale and then exhale as bring leg to chest, inhale as straighten leg.

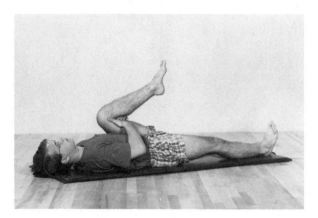

Figure 3.5. *One knee to chest*

Shoulder and Back Stretch at Wall or Ballet Barre

Benefits: Marvelous stretch for the spine, arms, shoulders and legs.

Precautions: None

Directions: Stand facing the wall, barre, or a counter top and have hands holding there as you back away so that feet are directly under the hips and apart, back is horizontal, arms are straight, neck is relaxed, shoulders are pulled toward spine. Feel the opening in the front of the chest, armpits, shoulders and a lengthening of the spine. You also may feel a stretch in the legs.

Breath: Breath normally.

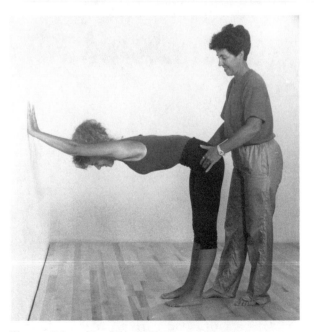

Figure 3.6. *Shoulder and back stretch at wall or ballet barre*

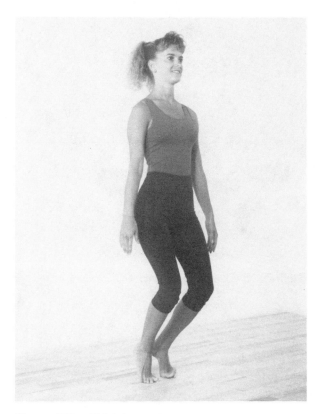

Figure 3.7.   *Thigh toner*

Thigh Toner

Benefits: Strengthens the quadriceps, muscles of feet and improves balance.
Precautions: Do not lower to far and cause stress on the knee.
Directions: Stand erect in good postural alignment and with toes spread raise on to them and balance as you lower body slightly. Hold as you count to 10 and then increase count.
Breath: Breath normally, there is a tendency to hold the breath.

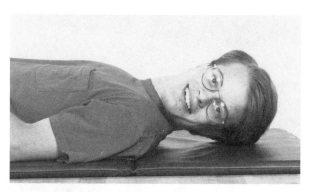

Figure 3.8.   *Head lift and turn*

Head Lift and Turn

Benefits: Strengthens muscles of the neck especially the sternocleidomastoid.
Precautions: Do not do if you have a recent neck injury.
Directions: Lying on back lift head an inch from the mat and hold for 6 counts, turn head to Right and hold for 6 counts, turn head to Left and hold for 6 counts, back to center and lower. Massage front of neck. Increase the count by 2 every lesson.
Breath: Do not hold -breath normally.

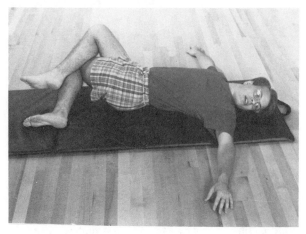

Figure 3.9.   *Knee overs*

Feldenkrais Kneeovers

Benefits: Gently stretches the muscles of rib cage, back, hips, chest and neck.
Precautions: Do gently, slowly and do not force any body parts- let gravity help.
Directions: Lie on your back with knees bent, Right leg over the Left and Left foot on floor, arms straight out to the side from the shoulder. Lower the legs to the Right and turn the head to the look at the Left hand. Hold. Switch the legs and repeat to the other side.
Breath: Take deep breaths and allow body to relax into the stretch.

Toe-Hold Leg Lift

Benefits: Improves flexibility of the knees, ankles and stretches hamstrings.

Precautions: Be careful if you have injured the hamstring.

Directions:
1. **With Necktie.** Sitting on mat bend knee and place necktie under the ball of the foot, holding ends of tie straighten leg and slowly raise the leg until a gentle stretch is felt. Hold and lower slowly and repeat with other leg.
2. **Holding Toes.** Bend knee and holding toe gently straighten the leg and bring the leg closer to the body without leaning back. When the stretch is felt hold at that position and gently lower the leg to the mat

Breath: Breath normally.

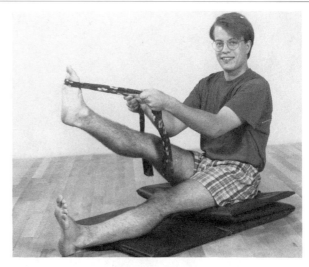

Figure 3.10a. *Toe-hold leg lift with necktie*

Alternate Leg Stretch
(Janusasana)

Benefits: Improves flexibility of the legs, back, and hip joint.

Precautions: Don't over stretch-go gently. Think of the muscles as rubberbands and control the stretch from beginning to end.

Directions:
1. **With necktie.** Sitting on mat with right leg extended slightly to the right and left leg bent with the sole of left foot next to the right thigh. Place necktie around the ball of the right foot and hold in both hands. With back erect, shoulders down from ears, lead with your sternum bringing chest closer to your right thigh. Do NOT drop head but gaze forward. Hold in your stretch. Repeat with the other leg.
2. Sitting in the same position as above. Place your hands on your shoulders and reach up straightening arms and lifting rib cage, contract abdominals and then move forward from the hip joint , head is up, shoulders away from the ears and then bring your hands down to the lower leg. Notice how the stretch feels in this position. If you want to increase the stretch move the hands closer to the feet. If you want to decrease the stretch move the hands closer to the knee. Hold and Repeat with other leg.

Breath: Inhale as you lift up lengthening the spine and exhale as you fold forward.

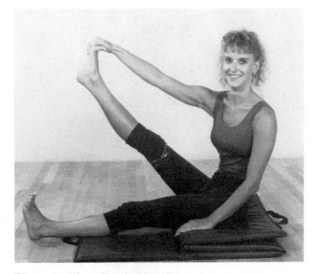

Figure 3.10b. *Toe-hold leg lift*

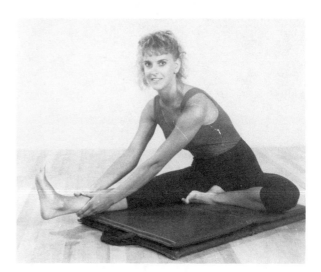

Figure 3.11. *Alternate leg stretch*

ASANAS

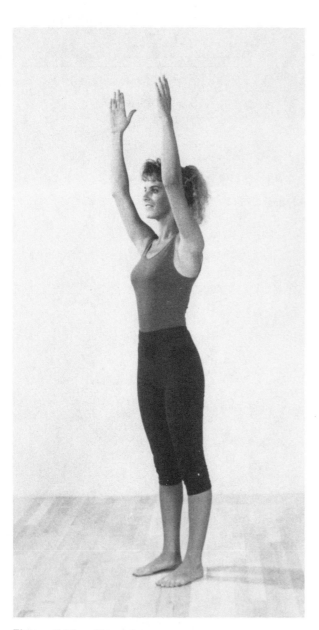

Figure 3.12.   *Mountain pose*

Mountain Pose (Tadasana)

Benefits: Improves posture and strengthens feet

Precautions: Don't lock the knees or allow the head to drop back.

Directions: Stand erect in bare feet, facing a mirror if possible. Legs are directly under the hips. Contract quadricep and abdominal muscles. Tuck the pelvis under and lift the chest. The head is balanced over the spine. Slowly raise the arms so they are pointing toward the ceiling, palms facing each other and fingers relaxed. Let the shoulders be relaxed and back.

Breath: Inhale deeply as the arms raise-the rib cage is also raising and can expand more. Breath full and deep while you hold the pose. Exhale as you lower the arms to your side.

Recommendations: When doing the mountain pose be aware of the strength of the feet and legs supporting you and a feeling of being "grounded" as a mountain is "grounded" in the earth. Also be aware of the lightness of the arms and rib cage as they are reaching up to the sky just as a mountain peak reaches into the clouds. Feel the spine lengthening. If you are working in front of a mirror check to see if the shoulders are level, the hips are level, feet both point straight ahead and that your weight is evenly placed on both feet. Standing sideways to a mirror check for an erect back with the shoulders not overly rounded (kyphosis) and the rear end protruding too much with a large curve in the lumbar spine (lordosis). The abdomen should be lifted. The head should not be forward of the spine as this increases the weight of the head and causes muscle fatigue. When you have the skeleton of the body lined up directly over the feet and the bones are bearing the weight as they are designed to there is a lot less work for the muscles, tendons and ligaments to do. Be aware at all times of your overall posture -whether you are standing or sitting. This standing position of the Mountain Pose is the base for all of the standing poses that will follow.

Cobra (Bhujangasana)

Benefits: Strengthens the muscles of the back and gently stretches the spine.

Precautions: Do not do if you have injured your spine recently. This is done slowly and with control. Do not put head back.

Directions: Lie on the abdomen with the hands placed under the shoulders, and the forehead resting on the mat. Move the head by brushing the chin across the mat, contract the abdominal muscles lifting the navel from the mat and slowly bring the chest up off the mat. Use the muscles of the back to lift with rather than pushing up with the arms. Keep the abdominal muscles engaged as you slowly lower the chest back to mat. Repeat twice.

Breath: Inhale as you lift up into the pose and exhale as you lower back to the mat.

Recommendations: This pose needs to be done with control and executed slowly. When in the pose the chin is lifted slightly and the gaze is slightly up - DO NOT put the head way back and compress the cervical vertebrae. The imagery here is of a snake moving slowly, with great flexibility and fluidity of movement. Don't hunch the shoulders by the ears and don't worry about straightening the arms. Be aware of the spine and the muscles of the back contracting. Always do a COUNTERPOSE of either the FETUS or KNEES TO CHEST pose.

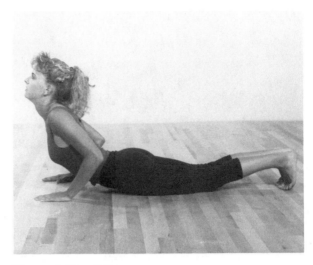

Figure 3.13. *Cobra*

Half Locust (Ardha Salabhasana)

Benefits: Strengthens muscles of back, rear end and legs.

Precautions: Do not do if you have injured or have a chronic problem with the lower back. If you have a problem with the sciatic nerve be cautious as you try this. Do the asana slowly and do not lift leg very high.

Directions: Lie on abdomen, with hands beside thighs, palms facing down. Place chin on the mat to keep the head straight. IMPORTANT: contract abdominal muscles-lifting the navel from the mat. Contract muscles of Right leg and lift leg slowly upward to the point you are comfortable. Hold and then lower with control. Do the Left leg and repeat 2 more times with each leg.

Breath: Inhale as you lift the leg and hold, Exhale as you lower.

Recommendations: Do not stay in pose too long and risk not being able to control the lowering. Always do the COUNTERPOSE of FETUS or KNEES TO CHEST.

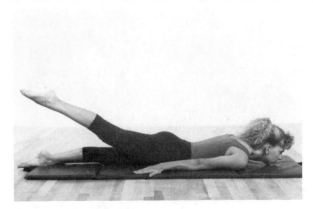

Figure 3.14. *Half-locust*

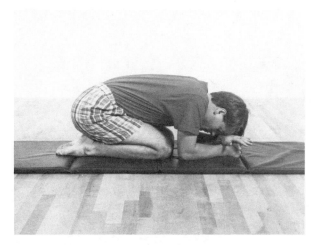

Figure 3.15a. *Fetus*

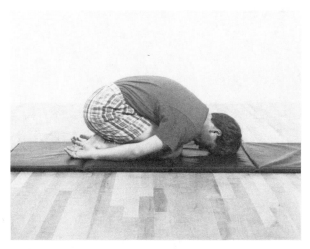

Figure 3.15b. *Fetus*

Fetus

Benefits: Is a gentle stretch for the entire back, relaxes the neck, improves flexibility in the legs, ankles and feet.

Precautions: May be uncomfortable if you have problems with injured knees or ankles. If so do the Knees to Chest pose following.

Directions: Kneeling, place hips on the heels and keep them there as you lower the head to the mat in several stages that will be described. If the hips leave the heels STOP at that position and rest in the pose. The head will be resting on the hands as they will change position-do the hand positions first:

1. Hands in fists one on top of the other
2. Top hand flattens out and is on top of bottom hand
3. Two hands make fists and go side by side
4. Two hands flatten -one on top of the other
5. Two hands slide apart to be side by side
6. Two hands slide clear apart for head to be on mat.
7. Move arms to rest on mat beside the legs allowing shoulders to fully relax

Breath: Breath normally as you relax and let go.

Recommendations: Always do this pose to gently stretch the muscles of the back after they have been contracted. Also do at any time when there is the feeling of tightness or fatigue in low back - such as after wearing high heels.

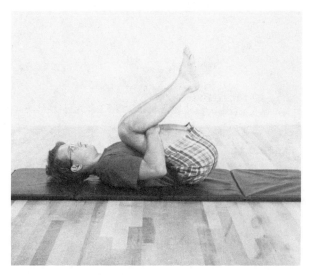

Figure 3.16. *Knees to chest*

Knees to Chest

Benefits: Gently stretches the back, and is an optional counterpose when the back muscles have been contracted.

Precautions: Do not place hands on lower legs.

Directions: Lie on back and bring both knees to chest with hands on thighs behind knees. Gently hug self feeling a gentle stretch on the back. Lifting head will increase the stretch.

Breath: Breath normally as you relax into stretch.

Recommendations: Do this pose when there is a problem with the knees or ankles that makes kneeling uncomfortable.

Sitting Forward Bend
(Paschimottansana)

Benefits: Improves flexibility of hamstrings, hips, back and lengthens spine.

Precautions: Don't overstretch.

Directions: Sitting with legs out straight in front of you and back erect, place necktie around ball of feet. Contract abdominals and bend forward at the hip joint - leading with the sternum and keeping the shoulders back and head up. Feel the stretch in the hamstrings and the back. Now bend the knees to take the stretch off the hamstrings and lower your self further feeling more stretch in the back. Repeat two more times.

Breath: Inhale as you lead with sternum and exhale as you fold forward at the hip joint. Breath normally as you relax into the stretch. Inhale as you lift up and exhale as you fold forward on your repeats.

Recommendations: Notice how far forward you moved into the pose before you felt the stretch so you can be aware of your progress. Notice also where you felt the tightness- legs or back. Do sideways to a mirror if possible to better note your progress. Also this pose can be done without the necktie when you have learned to keep a good alignment in the back- you place the hands on the lower legs, ankles or feet- where ever is comfortable.

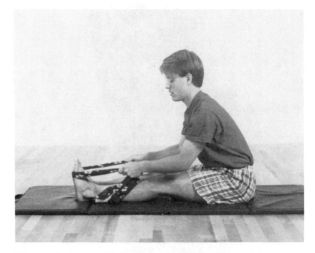

Figure 3.17a.   *Sitting forward bend with necktie*

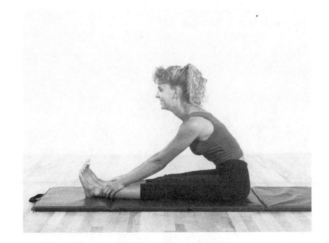

Figure 3.17b.   *Sitting forward bend*

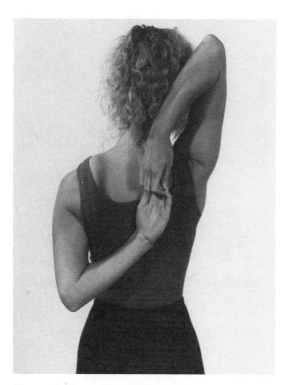

Figure 3.18a.   *Head of cow*

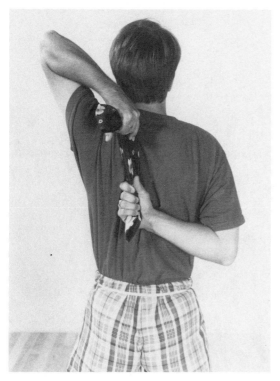

Figure 3.18b.   *Head of cow with necktie*

Head of Cow (Gomukhasana)

Benefits: Gently stretches the muscles of the shoulders, and arms and improves posture.

Precautions: Be cautious if you have injured your wrist, elbow or shoulder. Do not force yourself into the pose.

Directions: Stand erect, and raise right arm so the upper arm is by your ear and you can pat yourself on your back when you bend your elbow. Bring your left arm behind you with the palm facing out and placed as high on your back as you can reach. Now - Do Your hands touch? Can you join your fingers together? If so-congratulations! If not, use the necktie and drop it down your back with the right hand and grasp it with the left hand. Now that you are joined gently pull down with the left hand and gently pull up with the right hand and as you do so you will feel a gentle response in your arms and shoulders. Repeat, reversing arms.

Breath: Inhale and exhale normally. Do NOT hold breath.

Recommendations: Notice the ease in which you are able to join your hands or how far apart your hands are if you are using the neck tie. You may be able to do it on one side but not on the other. With daily practice you will make progress and be able to see and feel your improvement. A good time to practice is when you are showering and have the washcloth or towel to use in place of the necktie. Do not let anyone "HELP" you by pushing your hands closer together!. Look over your shoulder in a mirror to see your progress.

Chest Expansion
(Araha Chakrasana)

Benefits: Gently stretches the pectoral muscles, improves posture, prevents kyphosis (round shoulders), brings blood to face and brain, stretches out the muscles in the neck, improves flexibility of elbows and wrists and perks you up when feeling sluggish.

Precautions: Don't do if you have glaucoma or a problem with the retina of the eyes. If you have high or low blood pressure do not stay in the position with the head down very long and come up slowly.

Directions: Stand in the MOUNTAIN POSE (sideways to a mirror if possible),bring hands up to front of chest and extend arms straight out in front of you. Without allowing your trunk to move, separating the arms move them out to the side keeping them at shoulder height bringing the hands together and interlock the fingers behind you. STRAIGHTEN the arms and notice the marvelous stretch in front of chest. Now slowly bend forward allowing the arms to lift up and point toward ceiling. (If by a mirror- glance to see the arm position and how much space there is between your arms and your back.) With the head hanging free gently allow the head to make small circles, reverse the circles, and then come up slowly. Release the hands and enjoy the feeling of exhilaration! Repeat.

Breath: Inhale as you move arms back and Exhale as you bend forward and breath normally while you circle the head. Inhale as you come up and Exhale as you end pose and lower arms.

Recommendations: Always do slowly. If the stretch on the hamstrings is more than you are enjoying bend the knees. If you feel that you are getting dizzy- come up immediately but slowly.

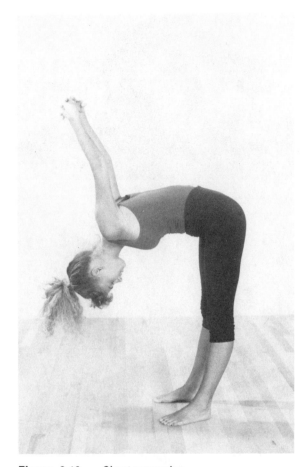

Figure 3.19. *Chest expansion*

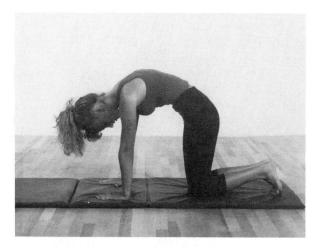

Figure 3.20a.   *Cat*

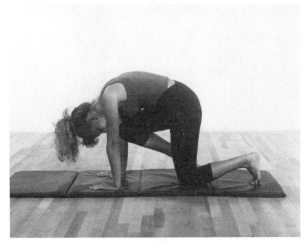

Figure 3.20b.   *Cat with knee in*

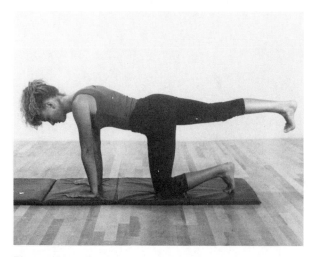

Figure 3.20c.   *Cat with leg extension*

Cat

Benefits: Improves flexibility of the back and hips.

Precautions: Knee problems can make kneeling uncomfortable. Have knees on a mat and hands on floor.

Directions: Kneeling (side to mirror if possible) place your palms, with fingers spread and pointing forward, directly under the shoulders, and have the inside of your elbows facing each other. Your knees are directly under the hips with space between them. Contract the abdominals. Lift your back up toward the ceiling like a cat and then lower until it sags. Repeat several times.

Variation: With Leg

As the back lifts bring a bent knee into the chest, as the back lowers extend the leg back so that the heel is in line with the buttocks and the shoulder, the foot is flexed and the head also lifts up and you gaze forward. Repeat with other leg and do two more with each leg.

Breath: Inhale and then Exhale as back lifts and/or knee comes in toward chest and then Inhale as head lifts and leg is extended.

Recommendations: Be aware of the abdominal area - don't let it sag. When the leg movement is added, do not let the heel be higher than the hip so the lumbar area of the back is not compressed. Be aware of the possible difference between the Right and Left leg as they come forward. Keep fingers flat and elbows in proper alignment. Shake your hands to release any tension in your wrists when you have finished.

Dog (Adho Mukha Svanasana)

Benefits: Improves flexibility in the legs, especially the gastrocnemius and shoulders, as well as lengthens the spine and strengthens the shoulders and arms. Is also an inverted pose which brings the blood to the face and brain and benefits that area without putting any strain on the muscles of the neck.

Precautions: Do not do if you have glaucoma or retina problems. Do not stay long if your have high or low blood pressure. If you have injured the achilles tendon be cautious when allowing the stretch to move into that area. *Must* be done in bare feet on the floor.

Directions: Starting position is the "all fours " used above in the CAT with all the same directions for achieving a good alignment. Adjust the hands to turn slightly inward about 1". Turn under the toes and grip with them and lift the buttocks toward the ceiling. Keep arms straight and press to floor with hands to better elongate the spine. BE STRONG. Lower your heels to the floor as far as you are comfortable. Bend your knees slightly and now lower your heels one at a time toward the floor. Lower your knees to the mat and release.

Breath: Inhale deeply before beginning and then keep the breath deep and regular as you hold in the pose. Do not hold the breath. The breath helps you stay energized to be strong in the pose.

Recommendations: Don't ever force. Think STRONG. Don't move the hands and feet from the starting alignment position. Do sideways to a mirror to see if you are achieving an upside down "V" position with the asana.

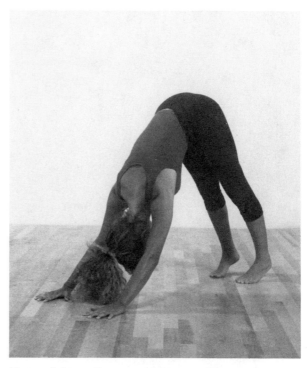

Figure 3.21. *Dog*

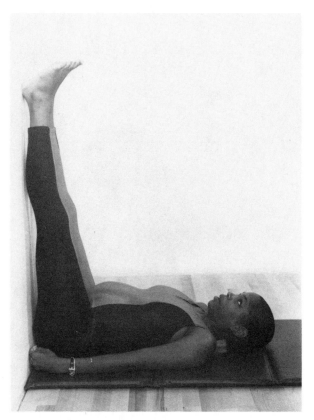

Figure 3.22a.   *Shoulderstand by the wall*

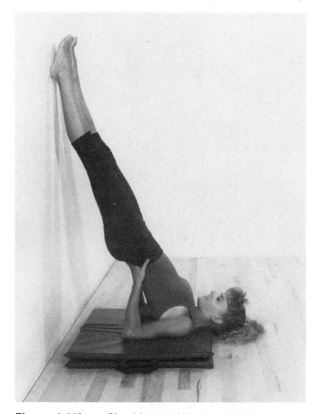

Figure 3.22b.   *Shoulderstand by the wall back lifted*

Shoulderstand (Sarvangasana)

Benefits: In Sanskrit the word Sarva means "all" and the word Anga means "parts". The name implies that this pose is for all body parts - thus there are many benefits. Being an inverted pose it allows the body to overcome some of the effects of gravity on the veins, arteries, and internal organs by placing the body in an opposite alignment. This can be helpful for a prolapsed uterus. The circulation to the legs, spine, thyroid gland and brain is enhanced by this pose. Those with asthma and throat problems are also benefitted by doing this pose. The muscles of the back and shoulders are strengthened. The pose is energizing.

Precautions: The major precautions will be discussed under the variations section as they will vary from one to the other. In general, though, this pose is not recommended for those with high blood pressure or recent neck injuries. If you are menstruating or are pregnant do the variation that is recommended below.

Directions: Will be given for each variation.

Variations:

A.   (see figure 3.22a) At the wall simply elevate the legs and be aware of the feeling in the legs as the circulation is affected by this position.

 Recommendations: This variation can be done by almost anyone. Especially should be done by those women who are pregnant or are having their menstrual cycle. This position is also safe for someone who has injured their neck, has high blood pressure, a hernia, or is 15-20 pounds overweight.

B.   (see figure 3.22b) By the wall with legs resting against the wall start to walk the feet up the wall and support the back with the hands. The body will now be in a slant with a little more weight up on the shoulders. Take one leg away from the wall at a time to get the feel for balancing. Then take both legs away and hold in a half shoulderstand position.

 Precautions: Do not do if pregnant.

 Recommendations: When you are feeling comfortable in this position you would be ready to work with the next variation. Remember this variation is not recommended if you are pregnant or menstruating. Follow with the FISH for your counterpose.

C.   **On Folded Blanket or Folded Yoga Mat** (see figure 3.22c) Fold either a solid blanket or a mat so it is about one to two inches thick. Lie on your mat with the edge of your shoulders about one inch away from the edge of the folded mat or blanket. Your head is resting on the floor and their is air or space between your cervical vertebra and the floor below. This allows the neck to maintain its natural curve and does not hyperextend the neck and the supporting muscles. It is nice to have a partner stand by your head to assist you with this alignment and to help guide you as you bring your knees to your chest, lift up your lower back and support it with your hands. Now that you are up you are ready to do some fine-tuning with your asana. Bring your shoulders toward the spine - squeezing them together. Slowly extend your legs up, tighten the buttocks and hamstrings and image that your spine is straight. Hold in the pose 1 to 2 minutes eventually working up to 4-5 minutes. Keep adjusting the rotation of the shoulder blades to the spine if you feel them losing the alignment. Remember to do the FISH.

Precautions: For this variation and the one following do <u>not</u> do if you are: pregnant, menstruating, have high blood pressure, a hernia, neck injury or are 15-20 pounds overweight your desirable weight. Also be careful if you are overtired or are recovering from an illness.

D - E. Leg movements: (see figures 3.22d and 3.22e) Do these when you are able to stay centered and balanced with back erect in VARIATION 3. The legs split apart in a wide V. Hold While the legs are in the V move them slowly from front to back allowing a gentle twist to happen stretching the back. Lower the Right toe to the floor behind your head and keep the Left foot reaching toward the ceiling. Lift the Right foot up and repeat with the Left going to floor behind the head. Place the soles of the feet together and draw the heels down toward the crotch with the knees out to the side. You will look like you are a frog!

Recommendations: Never turn your head, and always come down with control having your hands support your back until it is strong enough to uncurl. Keep the back of the head on the mat as you are rolling down out of the shoulderstand. Always do the COUNTER POSE of the FISH and the CHEST EXPANSION to balance the body. The feeling of fatigue in the back muscles will most likely disappear after the FISH and as you become stronger.

Breath: Keep the breath flowing at all times in all of the variations. As the abdominal muscles become stronger the feeling of pressure against your diaphragm will lessen. When you have come down out of your shoulderstand take some deep breaths.

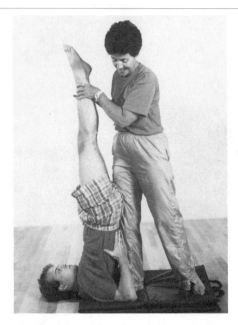

Figure 3.22c. *Shoulderstand on folded blanket or yoga mat*

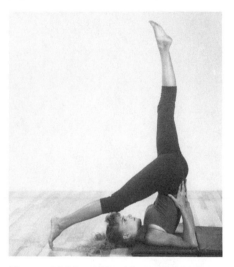

Figure 3.22d. *Shoulderstand with leg movements*

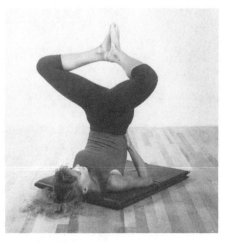

Figure 3.22e. *Shoulderstand with leg movements*

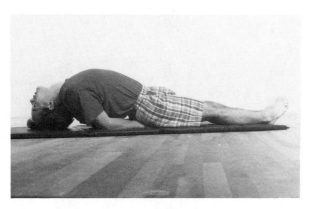

Figure 3.23.   *Fish*

Fish (Matsyasana)

Benefits: This pose is used as a counterpose to balance the body following the shoulderstand as it places the body in an opposite position. For example, the neck which had the chin to the chest is now being stretched with the head going back; the front of the chest was semi-cramped and in this pose it is opened up; and the back muscles were being strengthened and stretched and are now going to be contracted ridding you of any muscles tension you may be experiencing. It is also very beneficial for the nasal passages and the sinuses as the circulation is increased to the area and then when you raise the head you may notice drainage in the back of the throat.This pose also strengthens the muscles of the neck.

Precautions: Do not cough, swallow or sneeze in this position as your neck is in a vulnerable position. If you are susceptible to motion sickness or have an inner ear disturbance you may experience dizziness. If you have high blood pressure don't stay in the pose very long. This pose could also aggravate an old neck injury so be cautious as you try it your first time.

Directions: Lie on your back and place your hands, palm down, under your buttocks. Now raise up so that you are leaning back on your lower arms and elbows. Image lifting your sternum toward the ceiling and while maintaining the arch in your back slowly lean back until the top of the head is resting on the mat. Stay in this position for 4-5 deep breaths and as you exhale the last one lift the head up and sit up OR if the head feels very heavy (it actually weighs from 10-15 lbs.) slide your hands out from under you and lower back to the mat.

Breath: Inhale as deeply as you can through your nose allowing the chest to expand as fully as possible.

Recommendations: Do this pose daily if you are prone to nasal congestion or sinus problems. *Always* do following the SHOULDERSTAND.

Tree (Vriksasana)

Benefits: Strengthens the feet and the legs. Improves posture and balance, and flexibility of the hip and knee.

Precautions: May be challenging if you have injured your foot or ankle but don't be discouraged. To prevent falling out of balance do the pose placing a hand on a wall or chair back.

Directions: Begin by doing the MOUNTAIN POSE without the arm lift. Place the weight on the Left leg with the muscles contracted and holding you firm. Make small circle's with the Right leg before lifting it and placing the sole of the Right foot next to the inner Left thigh as high as you can take it and maintain the rest of the alignment suggestions AND your balance. The Right knee should be facing to the side. Now for the fine tuning: Tuck the pelvis under slightly-keep the hips level and the abdominal muscles contracted. If you are steady and balanced then start to make the arm movements: Slowly lift the arms above the head as you also lift the rib cage, but lower the shoulders, touch the fingers together with the elbows pointing to the side. Image a TREE that is solid with its roots in the earth and its upper branches light and reaching to the sky. With control lower the arms, then the Right leg. Pause and center in and then repeat with the weight on the Right leg and the Left leg lifted to the position. Be aware of any differences in balance, control or alignment between the two sides as you execute the asana.

Breath: The breath is very important in this posture. Inhale and then exhale as you make your movements. While holding in the pose breath deeply and keep the breath flowing so that you maintain energy and control.

Recommendations: It helps tremendously to FOCUS- on something that is not moving. Chose a spot on the floor or the wall in front of you. Try closing your eyes while in the TREE and see what happens. WHOOPS! Hope you didn't fall! Remember to be steady at one stage before you make your movement to the next position. This pose can be practiced while talking on the phone, doing dishes, washing face, standing in line- at least the leg position can be done.

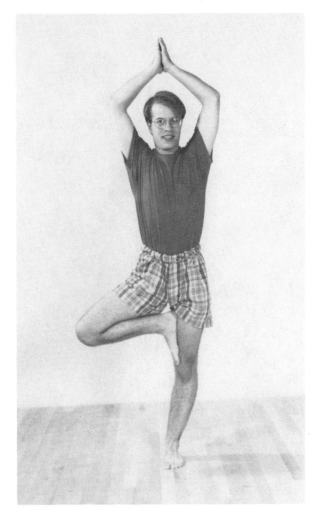

Figure 3.24.   *Tree*

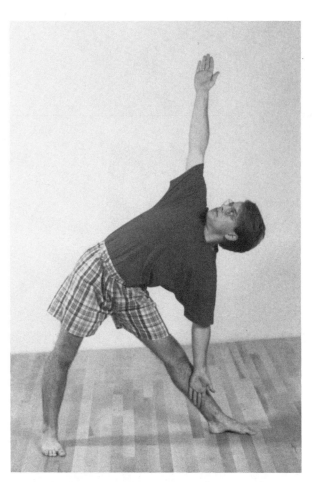

Figure 3.25.   *Triangle*

Triangle (Trikonasana)

Benefits: Improves flexibility of the spine and shoulders. Stretches the muscles of the leg and strengthens them also. Tone the muscles of the waist, abdomen and intercostal muscles of the ribcage which are so important for deep breathing.

Precautions: May notice fatigue in areas of old injuries such as shoulders, legs or back when doing the pose but this will go away as the area gains in strength. Stop if pain is present.

Directions: Stand in the MOUNTAIN POSE and then *jump* to a wide stance with the feet wider than the hips (3-4 ' apart). As you jump out extend your arms out to the side at shoulder height. Keep pelvis facing forward and arms level. IMPORTANT- pivot on the right heel rotating the femur outward in the hip joint and contract the quadricep muscles to stabalize the knee. Place the Right finger tips at the top of the Right thigh where the leg joins at the hip hinge and lean over to the Right side. Place the Right hand behind your head. Image that you are reaching to the far wall as you extend the arm out to the Right and lower your arm to rest in front of the Right knee but DON'T let the rib cage (which you extended) collapse. The Left arm is straight and pointing to the ceiling. Let the neck remain soft and when all the above has become automatic then turn your head to gaze upward at the hand. When you are coming up from the pose image that someone is holding your Left hand and is gently lifting you up to the beginning position. Pause and reflect on what you experienced and then repeat going to the Left side following all the above directions. Repeat 2 more times each side.

Breath: The breath is where you are going to get your energy to hold the asana. First Inhale deeply and Exhale as you jump to the straddle stance. Inhale as you turn the leg and then Exhale as you lower into the position. Breath deeply while holding in the asana. When ready to come up Inhale and then Exhale as you lift back to the beginning position. Inhale and Exhale here as you reflect and then Inhale as you turn the other leg and Exhale as you lower down to that side.

Recommendations: Remember to turn the foot to form a 90 degree angle with the arch of the other foot as this protects the knee. Practicing with your back to the wall helps you learn to keep your shoulders back and from rolling forward. Also it is helpful to practice in front of a mirror to check on the pelvis and the arm alignment. This pose must be done in bare feet.

Triangle Twist
(Parivritta Trikonasana)

Benefits: Same as for the TRIANGLE but as the spine rotates in this asana it increases the flexibility and strength of the back.

Precautions: Same as for the TRIANGLE except for adding a caution for those with a back injury that required fusion of the vertebra.

Directions: Jump into the pose as described in TRIANGLE, pivot on the heel also to turn the leg on the side that you will be moving to the Right. Now pivot at the waist turning to the Right and leading with your chest lean out over your leg. You will probably feel a stretch in the legs, but keep some of your weight on the back foot, your Left one. Twisting, place the Left hand on the Right leg. Notice where the hand is placed. You are feeling a stretch but not pain. Turn the head slightly so that you can gaze at the Right hand that is pointing to the ceiling with a straight arm. Pause and hold in the asana. Move the arms back until they are straight out from your shoulders, raise the trunk up and pivot back to face the front. Turn your feet to the front. Repeat all the moves now going to the Left side.

Breath: Pattern is the same as for the TRIANGLE. With the addition of the twist you may notice the chest being more cramped but as you are able to become more free in the pose the chest will be able to open up more. Keep the breath flowing while in the asana.

Recommendations: Always make sure that the quadriceps are contracted, foot is turned and the opposite hand goes down on the opposite leg in this asana. Don't lean on the leg. Don't over reach by going down to far on the leg and losing the twist. Walk around when finished and gently shake the legs to release any tension.

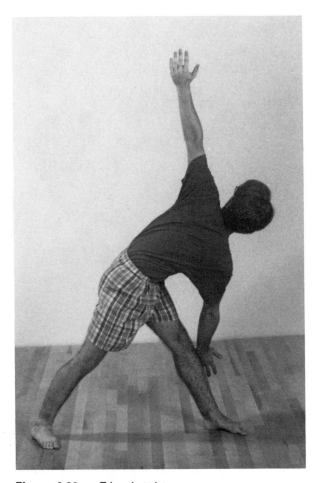

Figure 3.26.   *Triangle twist*

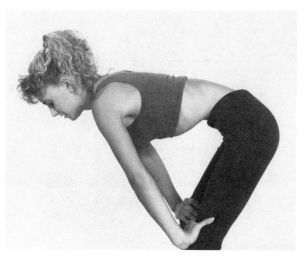

Figure 3.27.   *Abdominal lift*

Abdominal Lift (Uddiyana Bandha)

Benefits: This pose strengthens the abdominal muscles without putting any strain on the back. The circulation to the internal organs is increased and they are gently massaged. This pose is helpful for those who have a problem with constipation.

Precautions: Do not do this pose if you have: a full stomach, hernia, ulcer, recent abdominal surgery, or pregnant. If you have a "nervous stomach" do with caution and if you think causes discomfort STOP.

Directions & Breath: Stand with knees slightly bent and palms resting on thighs just above the knees. Take your Right hand and place on the abdomen so that you know what you are like there so that when you are doing the LIFT and you check you can make a comparison. Now EXHALE forcefully saying HA. Practice this several times and feel that you are emptying your lungs as you do this. Now the tricky part-with the air exhaled *contract and lift* the abdominal muscles toward the spine. Still holding, take your hand to feel your abdomen. Hopefully you can feel a change and that there is a "caved in" area where your abdomen used to be. If so you were quite successful for your first try. Don"t be discouraged as it takes practice to accomplish this but it is well worth the time spent. Hold the contraction for about 5-10 seconds and then release, stand up and take a deep breath before you repeat. Do this about 4-5 times and do daily.

Variation: Multiple Lifts

Once you have become proficient at doing the single ABDOMINAL LIFT you are ready to do this variation. When you have done your first abdominal contraction and with the breath in its suspended state you allow the muscles to lower but NOT relax and then contract them and lift abdomen back up and down as many times as you are comfortable with depending on your breath control. Don't do too many at first -3 or 4. The massage action is greater with this variation.

Recommendations: Practice these in the morning when the stomach is empty. It has been recommended to help with constipation to put 1 tsp. - 1 tbl. lemon juice in a glass of lukewarm water and drink this in the morning. Wait a few minutes for it to reach the stomach and then do the ABDOMINAL LIFT. This "wakes up" the digestive tract in a normal fashion. Also it is helpful to practice this pose in front of a mirror in your underwear so that you can see what is happening and better tune into your progress with this asana. It is recommended to do this pose following childbirth when the physician has said it is time to begin to exercise. This pose is an example of a BANDHA, a type of yoga position in which a lock is placed upon the body. We get the English word Bondage from this Sanskrit term.

Back Push-Up (Kamaharasana)

Benefits: This pose strengthens the buttocks, thighs, abdomen and pubococygeal muscle that is the base of abdominal area. Having strong the pubococygeal helps prevent incontinence. The flexibility of the spine and shoulders are also improved.

Precautions: Don't lift too high and hyperextend the neck.

Directions: The pelvic tilt will be taught as it is the first step in doing this asana. Lying on your back with knees bent and slightly apart, and feet flat on the floor and hands beside the hips. Contract the abdominals and feel the lumbar area of the back press into the mat. Now arch this area up away from the mat. Place one of your hands under this arched area and now tilt the pelvis down moving the back onto your hand. Arch up, take hand out and again do pelvic tilt pressing the lumbar area into the mat and contracting the abdominals as well. Now contract the muscles of the buttocks, thighs, abdominals and the pubococygeal (the muscle you tighten when you need to go to the bathroom and there isn't one available at that moment). Lift the buttocks and the rest of the back from the mat. Lift until you are on the shoulders, back of head and the feet. Slowly and with control lower the spine one vertebra after another. Now, we will add the arm movement- as the back lifts the arms will lift also until they are resting on the mat behind the head. Hold keeping the pelvis lifted. As you lower again do it slowly. Relax and take a deep breath.

Breath: Inhale as the back and the arms lift into the pose on a count of 6. Hold and breath normally and then Exhale as the back and arms lower to a count of 6.

Recommendations: As a counterpose do the KNEES TO CHEST to gently stretch out the spine. This asana is a preparation for the advanced asana of the Bridge and the Wheel.

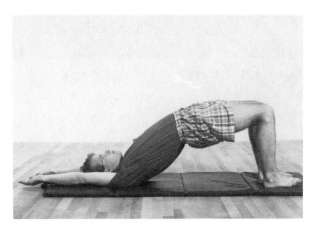

Figure 3.28. *Back push-up*

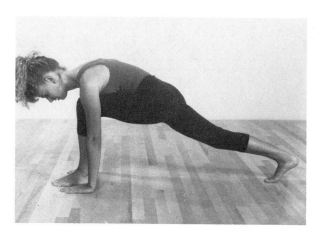

Figure 3.29.   *Lunge*

Lunge

Benefits: Improves the strength and flexibility of the legs, ankles and knees. Improves the flexibility of the pelvis.

Precautions: Go slowly if there are old injuries to the knee and ankle.

Directions: Do this pose with the side to the mirror if possible. Start standing and then bend the knees and place the palms on the floor beside the feet, lining up the toes and fingers. Take the weight on the Left foot and the hands as you place the Right leg back with the toes on the floor and then let the Right knee touch to the floor. There should be a stretch happening in the muscles of the thigh. Image that you are allowing the pelvis to sink toward the floor. The Left foot should be directly under the Left knee so that a right angle is formed at the knee and ankle joint. If it is not there move the foot forward or back to get this right angle. Lift the Right knee off the floor and raise the arms toward the ceiling. To end the pose place hands back on floor next to the feet and switch legs to do pose with Right leg forward and Left leg back.

Breath: Breath normally as you do the asana.

Recommendations: Make sure that the right angle at the knee and ankle is maintained. Allow relaxation to take place to facilitate the stretch.

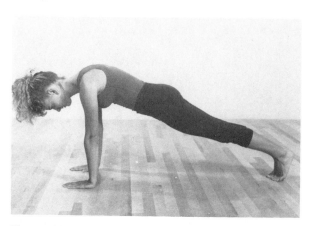

Figure 3.30.   *Plank*

Plank (Purvottasana)

Benefits: Muscles of the arms and shoulders are strengthened.

Precautions: Make sure you do this pose in bare feet so you don't slip. Be careful if you have old injuries to your arms or wrist.

Directions: Begin on all four's as in the CAT pose. Turn toes under and lift of the knees so that the body is straight like a board and weight is on the hands and toes. Rear end is down but back is not sagging. (similar to the up position in a push-up)

Breath: Inhale and then exhale as you lift off the knees, breath normally as you hold in the pose for about 6-10 sec. and then Exhale as you lower knees back to the floor.

Recommendations: Do this pose with your side to the mirror to check for straight alignment.

Lion

Benefits: Improves circulation to the throat and face. Tones the facial and throat muscles.

Precautions: Go slowly if you have a problem with the temporalmandibular joint.

Directions: Be prepared to be uninhibited when you do this pose. You may prefer to do it in private! Kneeling (or sitting) place your hands on your knees, lean forward slightly, stick your head forward, open your mouth as wide as you can, open your eyes as wide as you can and then stick out your tongue as far as it will go. You will look weird but it is fun to do!

Breath: You can exhale with a small roar if you want as you stick out the tongue.

Recommendations: This pose also warms up the vocal chords so it is recommended for singers. It also is helpful with sore throats that are caused by the irritation from post-nasal drip. Try it.

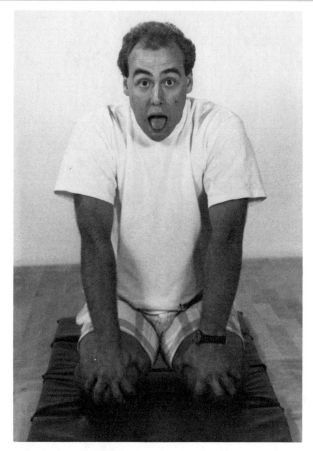

Figure 3.31. *Lion*

NOTE

The following group of hatha yoga poses may be more difficult or require more strength and flexibility to execute.

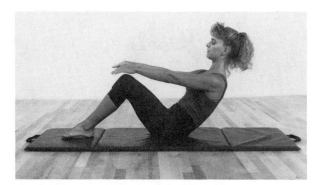

Figure 3.32a.   *Yoga sit back and up*

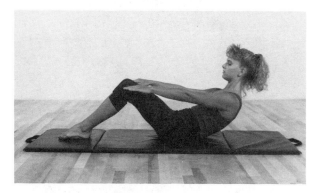

Figure 3.32b.   *Yoga sit back and up*

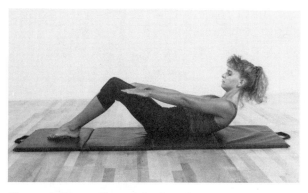

Figure 3.32c.   *Yoga sit back and up*

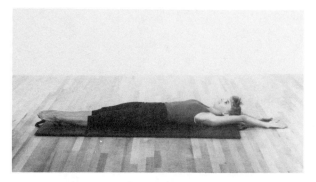

Figure 3.32d.   *Yoga sit back and up*

Yoga Sit Back and Up

Benefits: Can strengthen even very weak abdominal muscles in the sitting back phase.

Precautions: Could aggravate an injured tailbone or a hernia. Don't do immediately after abdominal surgery.

Directions: Do sitting on a mat with the back erect and knees bent. Contract the abdominal muscles firmly and while holding them contracted throughout the movement lower back 1) to a 45° angle and hold; 2) till you are on your sacrum and hold; 3) till you have the shoulders barely of the mat and hold;4) then release the contraction, stretch the arms and legs and take a deep breath. If you have strong abdominal muscles you will come up reversing the procedure. If your muscles are weak then roll over on to your side and repeat the going down phase.

Breath: Do not hold the breath. Breath shallowly in the top part of the lung when the abdomen is contracted.

Recommendations: Follow this pose with a gentle COBRA to gently stretch the abdominal muscles. Do this pose daily if your abdominal muscles are weak. Make sure you get a strong contraction before you move to the holding stages. Do 2-3 times. To increase the work load you can move the arms out to the side or above your head.

Spinal Twist
(Ardha Matsyendrasana)

Benefits: Improves greatly the flexibility of the spine. Makes you aware of your ability to turn equally to both sides. Gentle warm-up for all the muscles of the back.

Precautions: Do not do if you have a herniated disc. Be gentle with yourself if you have any other injuries to your back or neck. Improves breathing capacity.

Directions: Sit with back erect and both legs out straight in front of you. Bend the right leg placing the foot on the mat on the outside of the left knee with the right knee pointing toward the ceiling. Place your hands on top of the right knee and do a gentle turn to your right and to your left to warm up the back. Now lift the right arm upward, in an arc, and placing the palm on the floor behind the right buttock. The left arm is placed on the outside of the right thigh or knee applying some leverage as your head now turns to look over the right shoulder. Hold in the position as you count to 10. Turn slowly back to starting position and repeat with the twist going to the left.

Breath: You breath in a normal fashion in this pose. With the leg pressing next to the chest it is difficult to get a full deep breath as you are turning. Do NOT hold the breath- keep it flowing.

Recommendations: Keep the head level as it turns. Imagine the spine is a corkscrew and you are gradually turning the spine in that fashion as the twist progresses. Move your back hand to a new position if you feel you could twist further. Always remember that the opposite arm goes by the opposite leg for the maximum twist.

Variation: The leg that is out straight can be bent and the foot brought back under the opposite buttock. The arm by the leg can be straightened and the hand placed on the ankle. The arm that is back can be placed around waist. Eventually with practice the two hands can join under the bent knee.

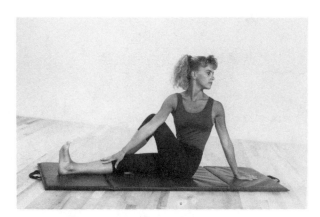

Figure 3.33a. *Spinal twist*

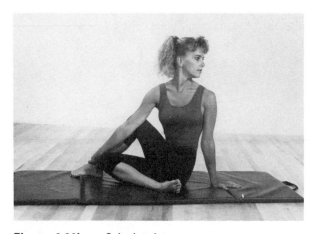

Figure 3.33b. *Spinal twist*

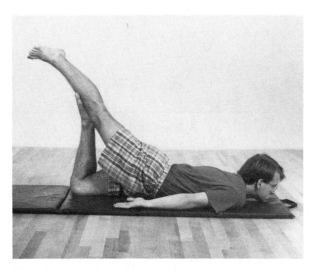

Figure 3.34.   *Flying locust*

Flying Locust

Benefits: Helps prepare the body for doing the full locust. Improves the strength and flexibility of the back. Strengthens the muscles of the buttocks and legs. Massages the uterus and intestines

Precautions: Do NOT do if you have injured the back, especially the lumbar area. Be gentle if you have had a problem with the sciatic nerve. Do Not do when you are pregnant.

Directions: Lying on abdomen, chin on the mat, arms are slightly under the body with fists under the thighs. Bend your left leg drawing the knee up to touch the fist. Contract the abdominal and gluteal muscles as you lift the straight right leg up and place it on the left foot. Relax, lower with control and repeat with left leg lifting.

Breath: Inhale and then lift the leg, exhale as you relax, breathing normal as you stay, and lower as you exhale.

Recommendations: Its important to keep the chin on the mat as that will keep the head straight and prevent a muscle spasm from developing in the neck area. Extend the leg that is lifted visualizing that you are lengthening it from the buttocks to the heel. Follow with the counterpose of the FETUS.

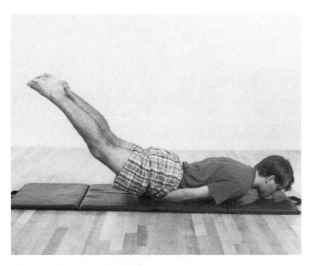

Figure 3.35.   *Full locust*

Full Locust (Salabhasana)

Benefits: Same as above but will strengthen more the muscles of the back, buttocks, and legs. Stimulates the circulation and endocrine systems.

Precautions: Those with high blood pressure, injuries to the back, herniated discs in lumbar area, heart ailments, or are pregnant should not do this pose.

Directions: You are lying on abdomen, chin on the mat, fists and arms are under the body so that your pelvis is resting on the arms. Gather your energy together, lift the muscles of the abdomen, tighten the muscles of the entire lower body, and LIFT both legs up. Keep the legs straight and stretching with toes pointed. Hold and then lower with control. Repeat 1-2 more.

Breath: Inhale as you lift up, and exhale as you lower your legs. Take a deep breath before repeating.

Recommendations: Do not try to kick up, as the momentum will just bring you back down. You need to squeeze the buttocks together and LIFT. Practice daily to maintain back strength and tone leg muscles.

Dolphin

Benefits: Brings blood to head, improving circulation to the brain. Strengthens arms, shoulders, and back. Stretches legs.

Precautions: Do not do if you have high blood pressure, glaucoma or retina problems.

Directions: Kneel on a mat with your forearms on the mat and the hands interlocked. Elbows should be directly under the shoulders. Move your knees back and then place the top of your head on the mat with the joined hands snug against the back of the head. Keep the shoulders lifted away from the ears so the neck is held strong. Straighten your legs lifting the buttocks toward the ceiling. Hold in this inverted position. Lower down and relax with the head on the mat. Repeat and this next time lift the head off the mat using the muscles of the back and the neck to do this. Hold noticing how the muscles are working to help you accomplish this. Do not allow the shoulders to collapse down on to the neck.

Breath: Breath normally as you attain the kneeling position. Then as you straighten the legs to lift the buttocks exhale. Inhale and exhale while maintaining the pose and then exhale when you lower buttocks down.

Recommendations: It is best to practice this after having down the CHEST EXPANSION, CAT and DOG poses. This pose is a preparation pose for the next one. (HEADSTAND HANG) You should be able to maintain the position with the head lifted for a count of ten with no fatigue before you proceed with the HEAD-STAND. Repeat it two or three times. Massage your neck, shoulders and arms when finished. This pose is good following childbirth.

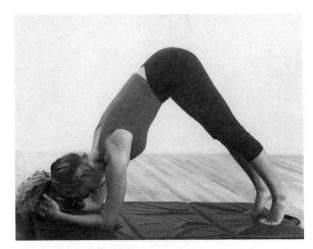

Figure 3.36.   *Dolphin*

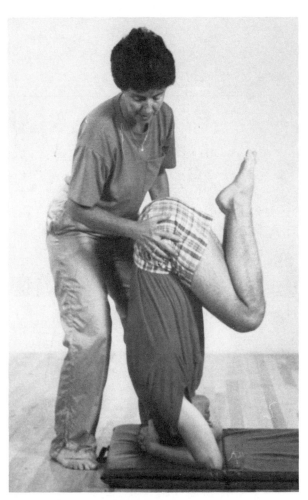

Figure 3.37.   *Headstand hang*

Headstand Hang
(Salamba Sirsaasana)

Benefits: This pose helps you gain confidence in your ability to balance your body in an inverted position without being afraid of falling. Again the circulation is benefitted by this inverted position. Internal organs are allowed to move into a position where the weight of other organs had been shifted from them.

Precautions: This pose should not be done by those with high blood pressure, glaucoma, retina problems, twenty pounds overweight, a neck injury or a hernia. Women do not do this pose during their menstrual cycle or when pregnant.

Directions: This pose requires a partner who will "spot" you. You will kneel down in the position described for the DOLPHIN and the partner will stand behind your head with one foot by your hands and the other foot by one elbow. Their leg will be behind your back when you are in the pose and their hands on your hips to help you become stable. Lift into the DOLPHIN and then walk your feet in toward your body. When you are as close as you can be then bend your knees bringing them to your chest and tilt the pelvis back slightly to find your center of balance. The partner can help by assisting with the lifting up and the centering of the pelvis. The hips will need to be back slightly toward their leg to counter balance the weight of the bent knees in the front. Partners do NOT let go of them but as you feel them become more centered and balanced you can lighten your touch until they can maintain the balance by themself. Hold for twenty to thirty seconds. Lower down with control by bringing the feet to the floor first, and then lower the knees. Keep the head on the mat while the partner massages your neck and shoulders. Lift up your head slowly so you don't get dizzy.

Breath: The breath is very important as it helps you maintain a sense of control and stability. You make all your moves as you EXHALE. You INHALE - then EXHALE as you lift up to the DOLPHIN; INHALE - then EXHALE as you walk your feet in; INHALE- then EXHALE as you bring the knees to your chest and balance. While in the HANG you breath normally. When you are ready to come down you INHALE- then EXHALE as you take your feet to the floor; INHALE- then EXHALE as you lower your knees to the mat; breath normally while you are being massaged. Doing the breathing in this manner assures your body of having the needed oxygen to do the pose.

Recommendations: Practice this with a partner to spot you. Keep the shoulders lifted up from the ears. Do NOT slump down on to the neck. If you are having trouble with tilting the pelvis to find your center of balance practice pelvic tilts lying on your back on the mat. Keep both elbows on the mat. Practice at this stage until you can easily maintain your balance without your partner holding you.

Headstand (Sirsasana)

Benefits: In addition to all the benefits mentioned for the DOLPHIN and the HANG, you will improve your posture and gain in self confidence when doing the HEADSTAND.

Precautions: Do not do if you have a neck injury, hernia, glaucoma, retina problems, are overweight, or have high blood pressure. Women should not do during their menstrual cycle or when pregnant.

Directions: Begin by doing the DOLPHIN, then move to the HANG and while your partner is stabilizing you at your hips you will straighten your legs. You will hold in the pose for 20 seconds to two minutes. When you are ready to come down do it slowly and with control using your breath. You will bend your knees to the chest and then lower the toes to the mat ending in the DOLPHIN. Lowering the hips down relax in the FETUS pose while the partner massages your back and shoulders.

Breath: The INHALE is done and then the movement of straightening the legs is done as you EXHALE. Breath normally and full as you maintain the pose and then EXHALE as you lower the legs.

Recommendation: To maintain your balance you need to contract the muscles of the quadriceps, and lengthen the muscles on the back of the thigh and calf. The abdominal, and buttock muscles are contracted as this helps keep the lower back from arching. Keeping the elbows under the shoulders also helps prevent the back from arching. The head should be straight so that the weight will be centered on a spot on the top of the head. To help find this spot put your index fingers on the top of your ears and move the fingers up until they meet on the top of the head. Bend down and place this area on the mat sliding the fingers away. When you are able to balance without the help of a spotter, practice by a wall. As you become stronger you will be able to go up with the legs straight. Don't stay too long, always maintain some energy to control your coming out of the headstand.

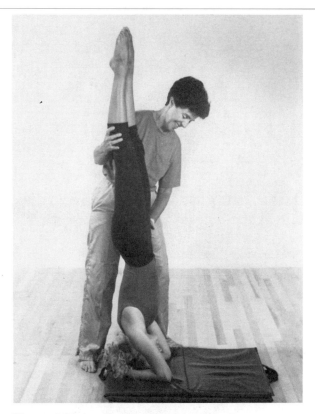

Figure 3.38a. *Headstand with spotter*

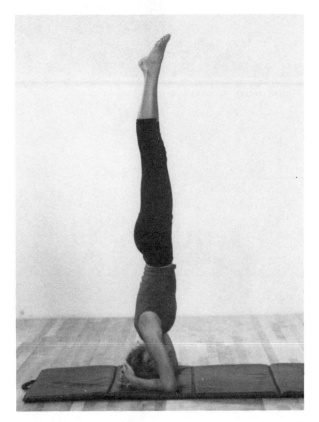

Figure 3.38b. *Headstand*

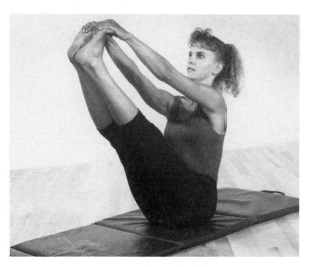

Figure 3.39a.   *Arrow sit*

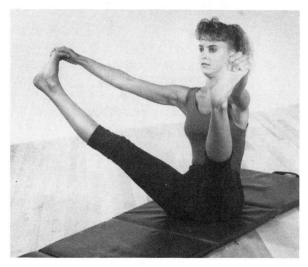

Figure 3.39b.   *Arrow sit*

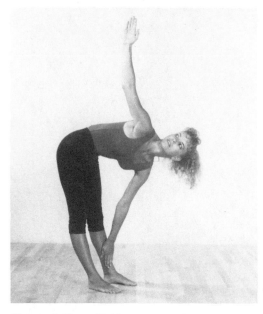

Figure 3.40.   *Rishi*

Arrow Sit
(Ubhaya Padangusthasana)

Benefits: Strengthens the abdominal muscles. Improves flexibility of legs.

Precautions: Maybe uncomfortable for a person who has injured their tailbone.

Directions: Sit with the knees bent and hands holding on to the toes. Lift the feet of the mat tilting back and balancing on your buttocks. Slowly straighten out your right leg and then your left leg. Balance and hold.

Breath: INHALE and then EXHALE as you make the movements.

Recommendations: Always do this on a mat or a padded surface. Do not force the legs straight if the hamstrings are tight. Make sure there is nothing behind you that you could hit your head on as you may roll back.

Rishi

Benefits: This pose balances and equalizes the sides of the body. You can also see the effects that Yoga poses have on the circulation system.

Precautions: Do not hold the pose very long if you have high blood pressure, or eye problems such as glaucoma or trouble with the retina.

Directions: Stand erect, lifting arms turn slowly to the right. Separate the arms placing the left hand on the inside of the left thigh and right arm is out to the right side. Slowly bend forward sliding the left hand down the left leg, bringing the right arm back so the spine is doing a twist and the right hand points to the ceiling. Keep the weight centered evenly on both feet. Lift up and bring the hands to the front and then repeat going to the left side. Do 2 more times on each side.

Breath: INHALE as you turn to the side and EXHALE as you bend forward. Breath normally as you are in the pose and then INHALE as you lift up and EXHALE as arms return to the front and lower.

Recommendations: This pose can stretch the hamstrings but if it is too intense bend the knees slightly.

Balance Posture (Natarajasana)

Benefits: Improves the balance, posture and stretches the leg that is lifted. Strengthens the support leg.

Precautions: May be a challenge for someone who has sprained their ankle or had a foot injury. Be careful if you have knee problems- use the necktie.

Directions: Standing erect bend the right leg and then reach down to hold the ankle or the foot with the right hand. The left arm is by the ear. Lean back slightly and then come forward allowing the right leg and arm to open up . Reach with the left arm and be strong with the left leg. With control move slowly back to your beginning position and lower leg and arm Repeat on the other side.

Breath: Keep breathing full and deep as it helps maintain the balance.

Recommendations: Focus on something as that will help you balance. This is a good preparation pose for the CAMEL.

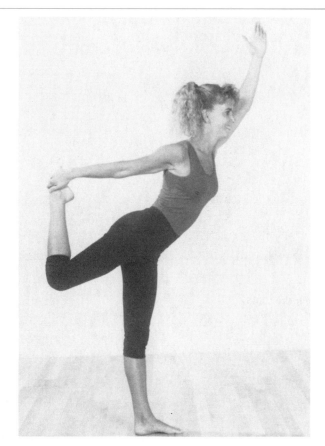

Figure 3.41.   *Balance posture*

Camel (Ustrasana)

Benefits: Improves the flexibility of the chest and spine. Strengthens thighs and neck muscles.

Precautions: Be careful if you have problems with your neck or low back. If kneeling on your knees causes you pain do not do.

Directions: Do a CHEST EXPANSION   and a BALANCE POSTURE as preparation poses. Kneel and then do the CHEST EXPANSION bringing the hands down to hold the heels. You push the pelvis forward as this helps keep the thighs perpendicular to the floor and over the knees. You lift the chest upward and allow the neck to stretch slightly but not dropping the head back. Lift up out of the pose and continue moving forward and down into the FETUS pose for a counterpose.

Breath: Inhale as you do the CHEST EXPANSION. Exhale as you move into the position. Breath normally as you hold.

Recommendations: Never do this without having done several preparation poses. Practice this facing a wall bringing the thighs to touch the wall. Always do a counter pose to stretch the back.

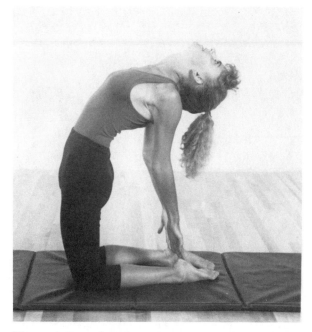

Figure 3.42.   *Camel*

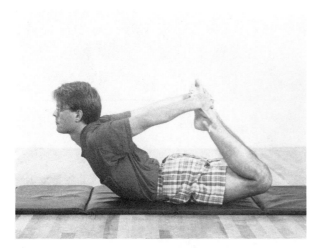

Figure 3.43.   *Bow*

Bow (Dhanurasana)

Benefits: Improves the flexibility of the back, shoulders, quadriceps and strengthens arms, and abdominal muscles. Massages the internal organs.

Precautions: Do not do if you have problems with the lower back or knees.

Directions: Lie on your abdomen, bend knees and reach back to hold the ankles or put a necktie around the ankles and hold the ends of the tie. With the thighs remaining on the mat lift the chest. With the chest remaining on the mat lift the legs so the thighs clear the mat. Now lift arms and legs from the mat. Arms are straight allowing the body to open up into the position. Hold and if comfortable rock back and forth slowly. Lower chest and legs with control. Repeat when you are ready.

Breath: Inhale as you reach back to take the ankles and exhale as you lift up. You will probably breath shallowly while on the abdomen.

Recommendations: Always do the fetus pose as a counterpose.

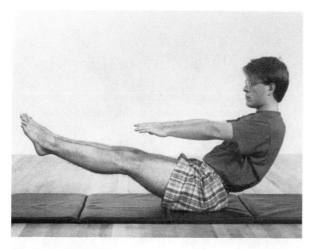

Figure 3.44.   *Boat*

Boat (Ardha Navasana)

Benefits: Strengthens the abdominal muscles and the legs.

Precautions: Could be an uncomfortable position for someone with an injured tailbone. Be careful if you have lower back problems.

Directions: Sit erect with the knees bent and arms crossed on the chest. Lean back slightly, lifting the feet from the floor and straighten the legs. Lower the legs until you are being challenged to maintain the pose and the abdominal muscles are strongly contracted and working. You can move the arms to make the pose more difficult - a) arms straight in front of you, b) arms out to the side, c) arms up over the head, d) hands clasped behind the head. Bend the knees and lower the feet. Repeat.

Breath: Breath normally as you are doing this pose. Do Not hold the breath as you are holding the legs out.

Recommendations: Make sure you practice this on a padded surface. If you think it could bother your back do NOT do.

Plough (Halasana)

Benefits: This pose is considered to be controversial. It can provide a nice stretch for the back and the legs. It also stimulates the glands in the neck.

Precautions: Do with caution if you have injured your neck or have a problem in the lower back.

Directions: This pose is going to be done with the head placed on the floor and the shoulders on the edge of the mat like the shoulder stand was taught. This prevents the hyperextension of the neck and allows the neck to maintain its natural curve. Lift up into a SHOULDER-STAND and then lower both straight legs toward the bench, wall, or the mat depending upon how flexible your hamstrings are. (Fig. 45). Placing the feet on the bench or wall takes some of the weight off the ligaments of the sacral area and does not overstretch and weaken this area. Hold for 20 seconds and lift back up to the shoulderstand and lower down out of the shoulderstand. Follow with a FISH as a counterpose.

Breath: INHALE and EXHALE as you lower the legs back. Breath normally while in the pose.

Recommendations: This pose should be done with caution and should not cause problems if done carefully and not held very long. Do not turn the head while in the PLOUGH.

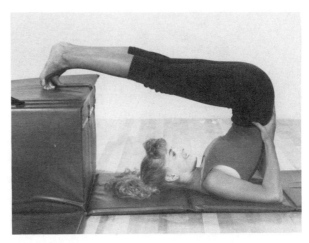

Figure 3.45. *Plough*

ROUTINES

Moon Salute

A popular form of practicing yoga is to do what are called "postural flows" or routines. This consists of doing a yoga pose and then moving smoothly to another pose using the breath to connect them. One of these known as the MOON SALUTE, (Fig. 3.46 on page 46) is a gentle stretching routine which moves the spine and improves the flexibility of the back.

Sun Salute

Another routine, one of the most popular and which has appeared in many magazines for fitness enthusiasts is the SUN SALUTE (Fig. 3.47 on page 47). The Sun Salute is a wonderful warm up routine improving flexibility of the spine and hips, and strengthening the arms. The whole body benefits from this routine.

Crocodile Routine

The CROCODILE ROUTINE of Swami Dev Murti, I learned in England at the International Yoga Centre which he established. This routine is done on the floor on a mat and consists of variations of the spinal twisting pose of the crocodile. When the body is horizontal the spine is free as gravity is then affecting each vertebrae and muscular area evenly. The routine is very gentle and helpful for anyone with back problems so if this applies to you refer to Unit 5 where it is presented in the section on Laughter (see Fig. 5.5 on page 65).

FIG. 3.46 A - L.   *Moon Salute*

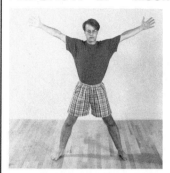

A.   Reach to Sky: Inhale. Arms reach overhead

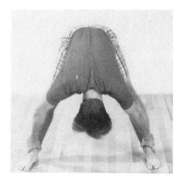

B.   Bow to Earth: Exhale. Move forward from hips, lowering arms with hands on lower legs, head hanging down relaxing neck.

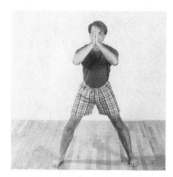

C.   Shooting Star: Inhale. Hands together in front of chest, straightening arms and looking up.

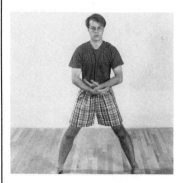

D.   Full Moon: Exhale. Lower arms making a large circle until hands are together one on top of the other by lower abdomen.

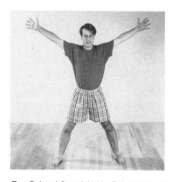

E.   Pointed Star: Inhale. Raise arms out to side with palms down.

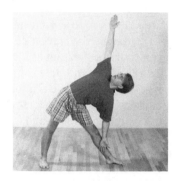

F.   Triangle: Exhale. Go to the Left side, following directions for figure 3.25.

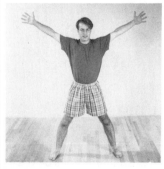

G.   Pointed Star: Inhale

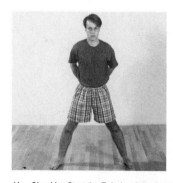

H.   Shoulder Stretch: Exhale. Arms behind you allowing the neck & shoulder to relax.

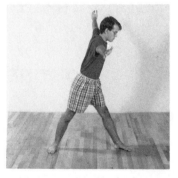

I.   Trunk Twist: Inhale. Turn trunk to Left side.

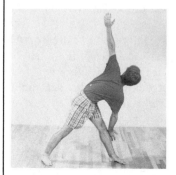

J.   Triangle Twist: Exhale. On Left side follow directions for figure 3.26.

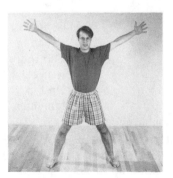

K.   Pointed Star: Inhale

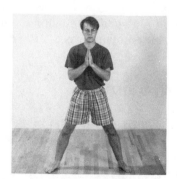

L.   End pose NAMASTE: Relax. Repeat going to the Right side for F,I, and J.

Figure 3.47 A - L.   *Salute to the Sun (Surya Namaskar)*

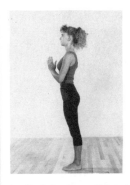

A. Beginning Pose: Exhale (see figure 3.12 on page 18)

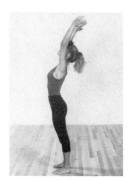

B. Slight Arch: Inhale. Tighten buttocks, lift rib cage and don't dorp head back.

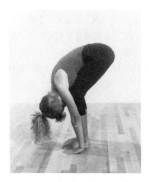

C. Standing Forward Bend. Exhale. Place hands beside feet.

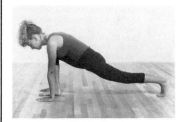

D. Lunge: Inhale. Take Right foot back. (see figure 3.29 on page 34)

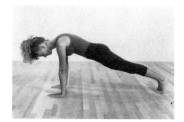

E. Plank: Hold the breath. (see figure 3.30 on page 34)

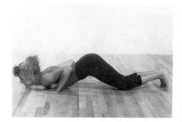

F. Knees & Chest: Exhale. Lower the knees to mat, chest between hands.

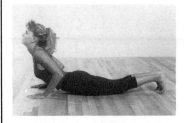

G. Cobra: Inhale. (see figure 3.13 on page 19)

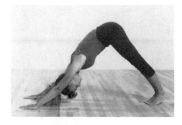

H. Dog: Exhale. (see figure 3.21 on page 25)

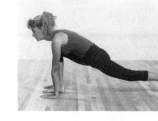

I. Lunge: Inhale. Bring Right foot up between hands. (see figure 3.29 on page 34)

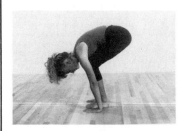

J Standing Forward Bend: Exhale. Bring Left leg up.

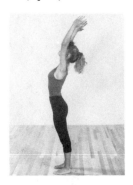

K. Slight Arch: Inhale. Tighten buttocks and lift rib cage.

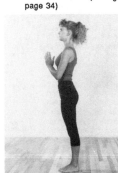

L. NAMASTE: Exhale. Hands together.

Repeat the routine again reversing the feet in the Lunge.

PARTNER YOGA

Doing PARTNER YOGA is great fun and a wonderful learning experience in working with and valuing another human. A partner can assist you in your stretching. It is important that you and the partner are close to the same size and have a similar level of flexibility. You need to be gentle with each other moving into the positions carefully. A sample partner yoga session follows in figure 3.48. Designate one of you Partner A and one of you Partner B and then follow the directions.

Figure 3.48 A - J.   *Partner Yoga*

A.   Knee-Thigh Stretch
Sitting erect with your backs touching "A" sits with the sole of the feet on the floor, knees bent and partner "B" has the soles of the feet touching and knees out to the side. Partner "A" reaches back and places the hands on partner "B's" thighs and gently exerts downward pressure until "A" says stop. Reverse positions.

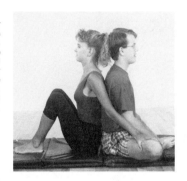

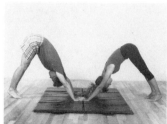

D.   Dog
Kneel down and sit back on your heels three feet away and facing your partner. Place your extended arms on the mat and interlock your fingers with your partner keep palms flat and shoulder distance apart. Sit back all the way on your heels, arms straight and forehead on the mat. Come up leaning to your RIGHT sides so now you are on your hands and knees. Turn your toes under, Inhale and lift the buttocks up so you are in the DOG pose. Exhale and move into a full stretch being anchored by your partners hands. Breath and Enjoy. Lower down and both relax in the FETUS pose.

B.   Spinal Twist
Sit facing with legs crossed at ankles and your knees touching and backs erect. Both place your LEFT arm behind your back and with your RIGHT arm reach around your partners RIGHT side to join hands with your partners LEFT hand. Keep heads and shoulders level and turn you head to the LEFT and gently pull on each other to twist more to the LEFT. Slowly turn back to facing each other. Repeat turning to the RIGHT with the LEFT arms around the partners LEFT side.

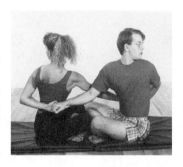

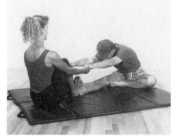

E.   Partner Alternate Leg Stretch
Partner "A" sits with the RIGHT leg straight and the sole of LEFT foot next to the inner right thigh. Partner "B" sits with the knees bent and the soles of the feet flexed against partners flexed RIGHT foot. Both INHALE. Lift chests and clasp hands or wrists, arms straight. Partner "B" gently draws "A" slightly forward with a straight spine and RIGHT leg. Hold at "A's" comfortable stretch and release slowly. Change legs and repeat. Relax and then reverse position for "B" to be stretched in this pose.

C.   Windmill-Triangle Twist
Stand back to back, with your feet 3-4 feet apart and about 1 foot away from the partner. Arms out to sides with hands lightly joined. Both turn to the SAME direction and pivot the heel of that foot to 90°. Lower the pair of arms on that side down and allow this pair of "Inside" arms to continue moving down passing between the bodies until the hands point to the ceiling. The "Outside" arms with the hands pivoting inside of each other have come down to the lower leg, ankle or floor depending upon the flexibility of the two of you. Reverse to come back up and repeat on the other side. Keep the legs straight and go slow to enjoy the stretching through each phase.

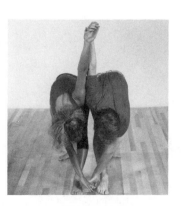

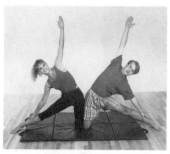

F.   Beam
Both kneel "thigh by thigh", with the outside leg out straight to the side, with toes pointing forward. Both raise arms and extend them upward. Inhale together and as you exhale lean to the outside with the outside arm lowered to rest hand on top of the lower leg. Inside arm follows the line of the trunk. Hold and breath normally. Exhale, lift up and reverse to repeat on the other side.

(continued)

Partner Yoga *(continued)*

G.   Chest Expansion
This is a very "trusting pose". Stand facing your partner four feet away with your own feet three to four feet apart. Place hands on hips and keep the hips over the feet concaving the lower back as you lean forward leading with the chest. Place the hands palm to palm and straighten the arms up toward the ceiling. The foreheads touch and the buttocks are pushed backward. The closer and more straight the arms are the greater the stretch in the pectorals. Release the hands slowly, straighten up, and massage each others shoulders.

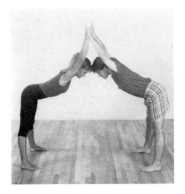

I.   Locust
(Do NOT do if you have back problems). Partner "A" lies prone with the hands on the floor by the thighs. Partner "B" stands by "A's" knees facing "A's" feet with her knees bent. Partner "A" lifts both legs and then "B" places hands under "A's" thighs and "B" straightens her legs to gently bring "A" into a higher position. Partner "B" should let the muscles of the thigh do the lifting NOT the back. "B" lower "A's" legs to the floor and then "A" rest in fetus pose while "B" massages "A's" back. Reverse and now "B" does the COBRA and the LOCUST.

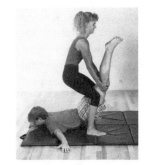

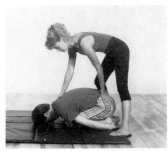

H.   Cobra
(Do NOT do if you have back problems). Partner "A" lies prone, clasps the hands behind the back as in the chest expansion position. Partner "B" kneels on each side of "A's" knees. Partner "A" lifts chest from floor as in the COBRA and then "B" takes "A's" clasped hands *gently* brings her further into the pose. Hold and lower slowly and do the next pose before reversing positions.

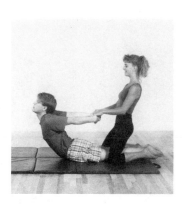

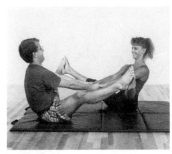

J.   Partner Arrow Sit
Sit facing each other, knees bent, heels on floor and toes pushing against partners toes. Join hands on the outside of the legs. Backs are erect. Slowly straighten up one pair of legs and then the other. Now without letting the feet and legs touch to the floor trade places with the arms so the legs are out in a wide "V" and the joined hands are now in the center. Lift the arms, bend the knees and return to the starting position. Repeat two more times.

BEGINNING YOGA PRACTICE SESSION

Do these routines whenever you want after you have learned the poses that are listed. Do each pose two - three times remembering to use your breath as it is taught when all of the basic instructions are presented. Always end with relaxation in the corpse pose.

Routine I

Neck Stretch and Turn (Figs. 3.1&2)
Body Rolls (Fig. 3.3)
Knee Thigh Stretch (Fig. 3.4)
Cobra (Fig. 3.13)
1/2 Locust (Fig. 3.14)
Fetus (Fig. 3.15)
Dog (Fig. 3.21)
Shoulder Stand (Fig. 3.22)
Fish (Fig. 3.23)
Triangle (Fig. 3.25)
Triangle Twist (Fig. 3.26)
Sitting Forward Bend (Fig. 3. 17)
Feldenkrais Kneeovers (Fig. 3.9)
Relaxation (Fig. 5. 2)

Routine II

Moon Salute (Fig. 3.46)
Thigh Toner (Fig. 3.7)
Sun Salute (Fig. 3.47)
Chest Expansion (Fig. 3.19)
Cat (Fig. 3.20)
Dog (Fig. 3.21)
Dolphin (Fig. 3.36)
Shoulder Stand (Fig. 3.22)
or Head Stand (Fig. 3.38)
Chest Expansion (Fig. 3.19)
Locust (Fig. 3.35)
Bow (Fig. 3.43)
Fetus (Fig. 3.15)
Feldenkrais Kneeovers (Fig. 3.9)
Relaxation (Fig. 5.2)

SUMMARY

This unit has the basics of the asanas taught in this book. Refer back to Unit 3 when you need to refresh your memory about a yoga pose and its directions, breathing pattern, benefits, precautions and recommendations. From now on the asanas will be referred to by their name and their figure number. Please read on for an explanation of the benefits of the yoga breathing techniques - Pranayama.

RESOURCES

Books
Folan, Lilias. *Lilias, Yoga, & Your Life.* New York, N.Y.: Macmillan Publishing Co., Inc. 1981.
Iyengar, B.K.S. *Light on Yoga.* New York, N.Y.: Schocken Books, 1965.
Smith, Bob. *Yoga For A New Age: A Modern Approach to Hatha Yoga.*
Englewood Cliffs, New Jersey.:Prentice-Hall, Inc. 1982.

Videos
Smith, Bob and Linda Smith. *Yoga with Breath Awareness.*
Lilias, Folan. *Lilias! Alive With Yoga.* Vol. 1, 2 and 3.

PRANAYAMA: Breathing Techniques

"Just as a child overcomes his clumsiness
by becoming aware of his body and learning to walk,
so does breath awareness gradually free the mind
from relating to the breath on an unconscious level
and this brings it under greater conscious control"
. . . John Clark- Foreward to *Science of Breath*

WHAT IS PRANAYAMA?

This aspect of yoga deals with the flow of energy, lifeforce or "Prana" through the body. Prana means energy and ayama means expansion. It is not only the breathing exercises but also the use of the life force within the physical body after the asanas have freed the body and the flow of the prana is enhanced. In Pranayama there is a conscious attempt to use the nose, throat, lungs, diaphragm, abdominal and intercostal muscles of the ribcage to direct the prana. Many times when we experience tension, sorrow or anger, we instinctively take a deep breath to calm ourselves or to gather more energy to see ourself through a difficult moment. In Yoga, the practice of pranayama is done with a conscious plan and is not left to instinct alone. Remember how the breath was a part of the execution of the asanas as they were taught in Unit 3? In this Unit the benefits and techniques of the complete breath, the alternate nostril, the Ha Breath with the abdominal lift, the Kapalabhati breath, and the bellows breath will be discussed. What research has discovered about the breath and recommendations for practice will also be presented.

Benefits

The following benefits are common to all of the types of yoga breath. The practioner learns to utilize the entire lung rather than only the upper portion which is the usual breath pattern. Also the muscles used in breathing are strengthened and the elasticity of the ribcage is maintained. Those with respiratory problems such as asthma, allergies, sinus or nasal congestion can be helped by practicing these breathing techniques. They are also recommended for coping with stress , to calm the body as well as to energize the body. Becoming aware of the breath and learning to control it leads to more respect for the importance of the respiratory system and how oxygen is needed by every cell in the body. This new awareness and concern for the health of their lungs has led some smokers to quit. Those in music and theater enjoy using these breathing techniques to enhance their control and ultimately their performance. Athletes also learn to value the breath control learned doing yoga.

Recommendations

How to position yourself? First of all be comfortable, loosen your clothing so there is nothing tight around your waist. You can sit in a chair or on the floor with the legs crossed in whatever position is the most comfortable for you. Try sitting with the pelvis elevated slightly (3-6 inches) as the back can now stay more erect and the hip joint and legs are more relaxed. Some of the breathing techniques will be done lying and some standing.

When to practice the breaths? This will vary with the type of breath you are wanting to do. When you wake up in the morning and before you get out of bed and again at night when you lie down are good times to do the complete breath as you already are in the position. Whenever you are feeling sluggish or tired during the day take some deep breaths to perk you up. When you need calming down use the breath to help you. Refer to

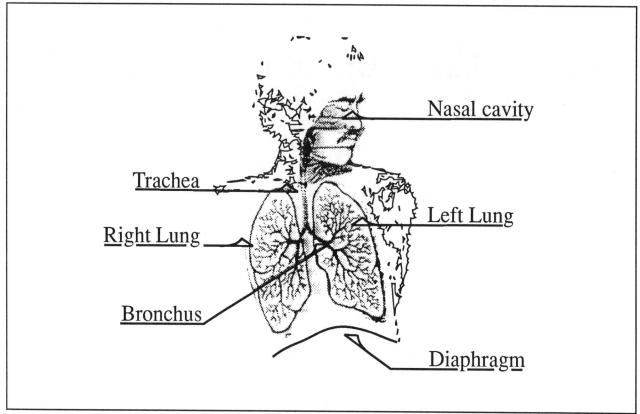

Figure 4.1.   *Respiratory System*

the diagram (Fig. 4.1) of the respiratory system to familiarize yourself with the area involved before you practice the following breathing techniques.

VARIETIES OF YOGA BREATHING

Complete Breath

Techniques

Position yourself in the corpse pose (Savasana in Unit 5). The Exhale begins with the diaphragm moving upward slightly to begin pushing the old air out. At the end of the exhale the abdominal and intercostal muscles will contract strongly. The abdomen will flatten and will continue to do so to empty the lung. The lower rib cage will squeeze inward. To add to your control with this breath you can use the throat muscles to assist you. Instead of "sniffing" the air in at the nose draw it in at the throat. When this is done correctly you will here a sound similar to a "small wheeze". You also are using the throat muscles to help control your exhalation and again there will be a sound. (Once you have learned this technique then use it for your breath that is done when you are doing the asanas. You will maintain your energy better for the execution of the asana.) Place your hands on the abdomen to monitor the lifting upwards of this area on the first phase of your breath, then move your hands so you can feel the ribs to monitor their movement outward as this part of the lungs begin to fill, and finally place your hands on the clavicles to monitor the upper part of the lungs filling. When you first begin to learn this breath the movements may be slight but don't be discouraged. With practice your body will follow your mental commands to breath in this fashion and eventually it will become a natural way for you to take a deep breath. When you exhale let your hands follow the areas as they return to their position when they were not involved in the complete breath.

Recommendations

1. Practice the breath several times daily and you will be calmer.
2. Do at night as it aids you in falling asleep.
3. Practice the breath lying on your abdomen as well so you can be more aware of the breath as the body is expanding and pressing downward at the abdomen and chest area.
4. Also it is very exciting to do the breath sitting back to back with a partner with the eyes closed. One does the complete breath and the other notices the feeling of the breath as it flows up and down their spine. This should be done after you both have been doing the breath for several weeks. This is very special as you are put in touch with this human in a way that is new to you both. You are "feeling" the life force within them and also noticing how the breath also takes place in the *back*.
5. Begin with a count of six for your inhale and six for your exhale. Work up to doing the breath for five minutes and gradually increase your time to fifteen minutes. Following your breathing stay in Savasana for at least ten minutes.

Ha Breath with Abdominal Lift

The basic instructions for this pose were presented in Unit 3 (p. 32) Practicing this breath brings you more in touch with your breathing muscles and strengthens them. This breath also prepares you to learn the KAPALABHATI and the BHASTRIKA breaths.

Alternate Nostril Breath
(Nadi Shadhanam)

This technique involves inhaling through one nostril, then exhaling through the other side; then inhaling on that side and exhaling through the nostril where you began (Fig. 4.2). To begin, you should be sitting with eyes closed, spine erect, and head centered and level. Place your index finger on the bridge of your nose, with the thumb

controlling the opening and closing of one nostril and the middle and ring finger controlling the other nostril. Check the flow of air in each nostril first, and begin the inhalation on the side that is most open. Inhale to a count of 4, 6, or 8 (whichever is most comfortable for your lung capacity), and exhale on the same count but through the other nostril. Then complete the round by inhaling on that side and exhaling on the side where you began. Repeat this cycle for a total of 6 times. Then take a normal deep breath and lie back or sit quietly to enjoy the calm feeling you have created for yourself.

There has been considerable research recently dealing with the connection between the breath and the brain. The yoga belief has been that the breath needs to occur in both nostrils to keep the body in balance and in sync. It has been discovered that the brains electrical activity can be stimulated in one hemisphere or the other depending on which nostril the breath is concentrated in. The breath in the right nostril activates the left hemisphere and the breath in the left nostril activates the right hemisphere as measured with an encephalogram. The autonomic nervous system and the hypothalamus have also been the subject of research using the breath. (see American Health, November 1986, p.16 & 18.) The exact connection between the nose and the mind is not clear at this point but hopefully science will find some answers to confirm what yogis have been doing for centuries.

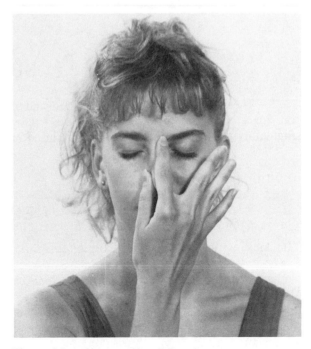

Figure 4.2. *Alternate Nostril Breath*

Kapalabhati

This breath involves a long, slow, controlled inhalation and a rapid, forceful exhalation contracting the diaphragm and abdominal muscles to empty the lungs. Repeat six more breaths allowing the inhalation to just happen but working on the exhalation. This breath helps the sinus passages to be cleared, also stimulates the internal organs and tones the abdominal muscles. Begin with seven breaths and gradually work up until you are doing twenty-one.

Bellows Breath (Bhastrika)

When doing this breath the abdominal area will function like a bellows that expands and contracts. This is a more powerful breath and should be learned after Kapalabhati has become an easy, naturally breath to perform.

The inhalation and exhalation are both vigorous and forceful, and one immediately follows the other. It is done more quickly than the other breaths. Do a total of seven gradually increasing the number until you are doing twenty-one.

This breath too clears the nasal passages and sinuses and also stimulates the entire abdominal area. This breath is not recommended for smokers as it may draw the residue of nicotine and tar deeper into the lungs. Don't do this breath if you are pregnant or have high blood pressure.

Master the known to find the unknown.
                    ...B.K.S. Iyengar

SUMMARY

These breathing techniques are tried and proven over centuries of practice by the yogis. It is well worth your time to practice them on your own to achieve the benefits that they have to offer from calming you to stimulating you and increasing the circulation. Refer to the resource listing for additional information.

RESOURCES

"In One Nostril , Out the Other", Brain/*Mind Bulletin,* August 1989.

Funderburk, James. Ph.D. *Science Studies Yoga: A Review of Physiological Data.,* Himalayan International Institute of Yoga Science and Philosophy, Honesdale, PA. 1977.

Miller, Richard. "Working with the Breath", *Yoga Journal,* September/October 1989. P. 67-75.

Rama, Swami. Rudolph Ballentine, M.D. and Alan Hymes, M.D. *Science of Breath: A Practical Guide,* Himalayan International Institute of Yoga Science and Philosophy, Honesdale, PA. 1979.

Shannahoff-Khalsa, David. "Breathing for the Brain", *American Health,* November, 1986. P. 16 and 18.

COPING WITH STRESS: Yoga Style

"There is a quiet, peaceful place,
deep down inside each and every one of us,
that can'tbe touched by the storms of life that swirl around us.
Learn how to become friends with your quiet, peaceful, inner self."
...Swami Rama, Founder of the Himalayan Institute
of Yoga Science and Philosophy

Yoga is recommended as an activity to help people cope with the stress in their life. As you will discover as you do yoga and read this unit it incorporates into its approach:

Exercise: which is always recommended for stress as it releases tension through physical activity.

Deep breathing: which was discussed in Unit 4.

Relaxation: which is done between the yoga asanas and at the end of a yoga session.

Imagery: which is also called visualization, which is done by having the mind use scenes of nature or of the inner body to bring about relaxation.

Music: which is used during relaxation to help with the freeing of the mind and body.

Meditation: which is taught based upon origins from yoga.

Each of these techniques, along with some others will be discussed in greater detail. First though a brief review of stress and its impact on the body.

STRESS

What Is It?

Stress was first identified by Hans Selye, a Hungarian who emigrated to the Unites States in 1931 and then on to Toronto, Canada. In 1936 he published his first article about his research with rats. When the rats had been deprived of their freedom and their diet was changed, they exhibited ulcerated stomachs and a loss of fat content in their thymus gland. (authors notes from Dr. Selye's lecture at Ball State University, 1979) His continued research over the years has resulted in his authoring 38 books and 1760 scientific articles. Now in one year there are over 6,000 reports made of stress research.

Dr. Selye defines stress as "the non specific response of the body to any demand". This means that good and bad events can both cause stress. The word "eustress" refers to a good event such as the excitement resulting from your team winning a close sporting event. "Distress" is the word used to describe the response from getting bad news about money or health. In both situations the body responds in a physical manner which is known as the "fight or flight response'. (Table 5.1) These are normal responses of the body to protect it from harm coming from a potential enemy. This response should not be thought of in only a negative manner as it can

Table 5.1. *Fight or Flight Response*	
Breathing speeds up	Heart rate increases
Perspiration increases	Pupils dilate
Blood pressure raises	Muscles in arms and
Digestion stops	legs tense
Body can begin	Blood goes to muscles
shaking	Feel restless
Feel keyed up	

function as a force that brings about a desire to create and accomplish a goal. We can let our incentive and growth be enhanced if we think of stress with this attitude. However when the level of stress remains high for an extended period of time, the body can develop some disorders that can lead to health problems (Table 5.2)

Dr. Selye thinks that there is a certain amount of energy available for our use throughout our life and that when this is used up we reach a stage of exhaustion and eventually die. Stress affects this level of resistance. He calls this concept the "General Adaptation Syndrone." The important thing to remember is that we can change the length of time that we stay in the "stage of resistance" by doing some stress coping activities, thus preserving some of our life energy and not reaching "exhaustion stage" where the disorders begin showing up. In beginning to cope with stress it is important to be aware of your response to the stressor. You are in charge of this response and how you perceive an event that causes stress. You are responsible for your own emotional and physical response. Your perception of the event is under your control even if the event is not. Stress of one kind or another will always be with you so what can be of help is to 1) identify what *causes* the stress for you by referring to the checklists in unit two 2) discover effective ways to alleviate the stress by reading the next section.

Table 5.2. *Some Stress-Related Disorders*
Accidents
Acne
Alcoholism
Allergies
Asthma
Backache
Chronic fatigue
Coronary Artery Disease
Depression
Duodenal ulcer/colitis
Eczema
Heartburn
Hypertension
Migraine headaches
Nervous tics
Obesity
Sexual dysfunction in both men and women
Spastic colon

WHAT CAN I DO TO HELP COPE WITH STRESS?

Physical Activity and Relaxation

Dr. Selye has suggested that the person who exercises regularly is able to resist the stressors in their life. Hatha Yoga poses are ideal for this as they do not increase the stress on the body as some forms of exercise can do for some people. The yoga stretches have been referred to as "Mother Nature's tranquilizer"- to stretch a muscle helps relax a muscle.

When doing yoga asanas you are encouraged to work while you are doing the pose and then to" let go" when you have completed the exercise allowing the body to go limp. You should feel the energy and thrill of the *doing* of the asana and then feel the *release* of the tension as you allow yourself to relax between the asanas.

In yoga we do the complete relaxation pose, Savasana, In English Sava means "corpse" and you want the body to be as free of tension as it would be if it were a corpse. In India the belief in reincarnation is popular so their using the corpse for imagery is not upsetting to them. Our western minds are sometimes not as comfortable with this image so it is sometimes referred to as the "sponge" or as the "yoga relaxation pose".

There are at least a couple of ways to reach this relaxed state. One technique involves tensing a body part before giving it the cue to relax. Another approach is to talk to the body giving it the cues with no tensing of the area. Both approaches work and it is usually a matter of personal preference and or time as to which method is used. Refer to Fig. 5.2 and follow these directions to achieve a stress free alignment for the body in Savasana, the corpse pose as it is known in English.

SAVASANA; Sitting with the knees bent, place your two fists between your knees. Now look down and make sure your feet are a little wider than your knees. Put your hands on top of your knees. Straighten your right leg, straighten out your left leg so they form the letter "V". Slowly , as you lower your back to the mat, imagine that you are placing each vertebrae down one after the other. You are laying the spine on the floor as you would lay down a row of blocks. Now bend your elbows, bring your fingertips up to touch the shoulders. Place the elbows in next to your ribs and then slide them out about

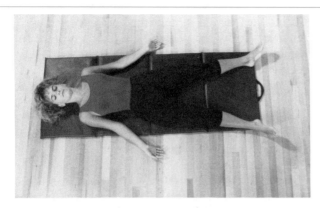

Figure 5.2. *Savasana*

3-4 inches. Straighten out your arms, bringing the lower arms down so that the palms are turned UP to the ceiling and you have your shoulderblades tucked slightly together. Now you are in your yoga relaxation position. Palms must be turned up. If the palms are turned down you feel your shoulders leave the mat. Following are some adjustments you can make for greater comfort. If you have a lower back problem and it bothers your back to lie with your legs straight, bend your knees or place a pillow under your legs. If you are feeling tension in the neck or shoulders turn your head slowly from side to side. When you bring it back to the center, line up the nose, chin and sternum.

Now that the body is correctly positioned, you want to be aware of your breath and allow the body to totally relax. If you are feeling tension in an area take a moment to gently suggest mentally for that part of you to relax. Also suggest to your mind to relax by being aware of your breath or the relaxation music that may be playing.

At the end of your relaxation time follow these directions. Keeping the eyes closed, lift your arms up as you inhale, hook your thumbs together and stretch the arms over your head and on to the floor behind you. Turn onto your right side. and move the body into a half moon with the arms and legs behind you, stretching the abdominal area. Then release that stretch and roll onto your back. Turn onto your left side and arch and stretch. Release. Bend your knees, with your feet flat on the mat tilt the pelvis and then turn onto your right side. Place the left arm across your body, palm to the floor in front of the chest. Bend your right elbow slightly, then using your two hands slowly push yourself up to a sitting position on the right thigh. Eyes are still closed. Sit with your legs crossed at the ankles and the

back erect. Now comes the "palming technique". Take your hands and rub them together until they are nice and hot and place the palms over your eyes. Open your eyes, slide the fingers apart to let in a little light and bring your hands down. This is a gentler way to reenter the environment.

Pranayama

Unit 4 discussed the benefits and directions for yoga breathing. It is again mentioned here as a reminder that the breath has a calming effect on the body and can be practiced as a stress coping technique. While lying in the relaxation pose described above practice the Yoga Complete Breath. Allow the entire chest and abdominal area to expand as you slowly inhale and then slowly control the exhale. Before meditation do the Alternate Nostril Breath. All of the Pranayama techniques taught are beneficial.

Meditation

What is meditation? It has been made to seem rather mysterious and sometimes controversial. It actually involves sitting quietly, allowing the body to become calm, taking deep breaths and allowing the mind to be still. Throughout history and in all parts of the world there are examples of "Meditation." It is not something new that came out of the "hippy era". It can take the form of a simple prayer or of sitting alone on a beach watching the ocean or on a mountaintop watching clouds.

Meditation was practiced; by the early Christian monks who were hermits living in the desert in the fourth century; in the ancient Jewish tradition where the teachings of meditation were called Kabbalah; by the Moslems who also have a tradition of meditation; in the Hindu method which has been taught to many westerners (Beatles included) by Maharishi Mahish Yogi and is known as TM - Trancendental Meditation; by Tibetan Buddhists and there is also the Zen tradition from Japan. All of these approachs differ somewhat in their technique but the end result is similar in that the stilling of the body leads to the calming of the mind.

It is difficult to describe what can happen as everyone responds to meditation in their own way and develops a technique at their own pace. It is probably close to being asleep but at the same time being aware of your surroundings-you are in what is called the alpha state.

Following are some suggestions for meditating following the hatha yoga asanas, relaxation and pranayama:

1. Sit with hips elevated on a small pillow with the legs crossed, back erect, hands resting on the knees, eyes closed and head level.
2. Allow the mind to be quiet- forget the past, present, and the future.
3. Regulate your breath for 5 minutes exhale on a count of 3-4 and inhale on a count of 3-4.
4. Allow the mind to wander for awhile. Do not FORCE it to be still.
5. Focus on your breath or on a word that you like such as LOVE, PEACE, JOY or the Sanskrit word OHM.
6. You can also focus between your eyebrows at the "minds eye" or at the heart center.
7. Stay calm and don't force yourself. ENJOY
8. 20 minutes is fine but longer is all right too.

Biofeedback

The definition of this word, simply means that the signals from your own body are listened to by YOU. In 1970 scientists at the Menninger Foundation Research Department in Topeka, Kansas collaborated with Swami Rama, a yoga teacher from India. He was asked to serve a year as a consultant to their Voluntary Controls Project. Here he domonstrated precise control over his autonomic nervous system and brain. The findings of this research increased the understanding of the humans' ability to develop this control for themselves. This led to the development of electronic machines that inform a person when they are developing the technique of tuning in to themselves. These machines and hand held thermometers are used now by physical therapists, counsellors and psychologists, dentists and nurses to help in treatment. The following are conditions where biofeedback is being used: migraine and tension headaches, epilepsy, cardiac arrhythmias, high and low blood pressure, paralysis and other movement disorders and digestive tract problems. The basic step in using biofeedback is doing the relaxation that allows the "Fight or Flight" responses to abate. It is thought that biofeedback works because the patient knows they are relaxed by the information they receive from the machine about the change in skin temperature or muscle tension. The signal received is like a reward for having achieved the relaxed state and they received the "feed back". When doing yoga with awareness and breath you are training yourself to develop this feedback system internally. If you should need biofeedback training to help you through a health situation refer to the Resources section for address of who to contact.

It is interesting to know that at the Himalayan Institute in Honesdale, PA. established by Swami Rama in the 1970's, they now offer a Biofeedback profile to let people know how well they are doing their yoga breath and relaxation. We have come full circle as the Biofeedback machines are now giving "Feedback" to yoga practioners. Instruction to improve your breathing and relaxation is then available if desired.

Music

One of the researchers in the use of music to lower stress was Steve Halpern, Ph.D. , who as a musician and a composer noticed changes in himself when he played the trumpet and guitar in his jazz fusion band and when after meditating he played the piano freestyle; what ever came out flowing, gentle music, with no beat. Since his first interest in 1969 he has become one of the leaders in the growth of "New Age Music". "My work has shown me that music can be not only a source of pleasure and entertainment but also a tool for reducing stress and improving our well being. In fact we can create music specifically aimed at making our lives balanced and peaceful." (The 1989 Guide to New Age Living, p. 62-64. Musical Meditation by Steve Halpern)

He returned to graduate school at Sonoma State University and conducted research using his compositions and classical music, measuring subjects responses to each by using Kirlian photography (high frequency, high voltage electrophotography developed by the Russians that produced a picture of the energy field that surrounds the physical body the "Aura"); electroencephalogram (measuring brain waves); and Galvanic skin response (electrical resistance on the surface of the the skin). No matter what technique was used the music of Steve Halpern produced a "statistically significant" effect on a wide variety of subjects. For example the brain waves would be in the beta range (13-39 cycles per second) for classical music and in the alpha range (8-12 cycles per second) for the new age music.

As reported in the book Healthy Pleasures, by Robert Ornstein Ph.D. and David Sobel, M.D., research conducted in California, Japan and West Germany has led to discoveries that indicate:

- music stimulates the release of endorphins, the opiate-like chemicals that the brain produces.
- that the beat of the music will cause the heart to speed up or slow down
- the electrical rhythms of the brain are also altered
- slower, quiet music with no singing lowers blood pressure and respiration
- soothing music played before, during and after surgery in operating rooms reduces the level of stress hormones in the blood
- music played in coronary care units reduced heart rates, lowered blood pressure, lessened depression and increased tolerance for pain
- during childbirth among women trained in the Lamaze technique music reduced pain and shortened labor by two hours.
- Music therapy may be helpful with autistic children, coma patients, cancer, stroke, arthritic and diabetic patients and premature infants.
- in healthy people it is thought that the function of the immune system is enhanced by music.

There are many individuals who have contributed to this growing field of music therapy by composing music and combining sounds from nature with musical instruments to produce this "New Age " music or "Space Music" as it is sometimes refered to. It is most often in a yoga class or a massage session that people are first exposed to this wonderful music that facilitates greatly a state of relaxation. Consult the Resource list for names and addresses for obtaining this music. There are publications that discuss this type of music and the artists performing it.

Imagery and Visualization

When you are relaxing in the yoga pose of Savasana (corpse) it is a good time to do some visualization. You can create in your mind's eye a beautiful setting in nature such as a mountain top, under your favorite tree or by the ocean, allowing your mind to recreate the sounds, sights, feel of the breeze, warmth of the sun, smell of the ocean, flowers or a pine tree. This will have a calming effect on you and will allow your mind to center in on this pleasant task. Then it can not think of your other concerns or problems.

This connection between the brain and the body is becoming more widely recognized. It is being discussed in popular magazines and also researched in respected centers of learning such as Harvard, Yale, and Duke Universities. The applications of this emerging field of study range from simply practicing positive thinking to the intense mental practice used by Olympic athletes to perfect their skills. It is recommended that whenever you could benefit from this imagery or mental practice in your daily life you should allow some time to develop this technique. Perhaps it may involve learning a new skill such as typing or the use of computers, or a sports skill such as your tennis or golf swing. This technique is also part of the approach taken in the many self-healing programs and books that have appeared in recent years. Dr. Carl Simonton and his wife Stephanie Matthews Simonton, Bernard Siegal M.D., and Norman Cousins have all made use of this approach and similar ones to help people in situations of chronic pain and terminal illness. They all have written books that are listed in the Resources at the end of the unit.

To further the study of the mind/body in a scientific manner, the Institute for the Advancement of Health was established in 1983. The institute, which is headed by Eileen Rockefeller Gowald, publishes a scholarly journal, *Advances,* and funds research projects dealing with the brain and immune system interactions; stress and health; and behavioral and psychological treatments for medical disorders. An astronaut from the Apollo 14 flight to the moon, Edgar Mitchell, has founded a non-profit organization, Institue of Noetic Sciences, that also funds research projects in this emerging field of psychoneuroimmunology. (See Resources) The future will undoubtedly bring further findings and a greater understanding of this complicated and important mind/body connection.

Chakras

One of the branches of yoga that is known as Kundalini deals with the flow of the energy through the body. There are seven chakras beginning at the base of the spine, #1, and ending at the crown of the head, #7. It is thought that these energy centers correspond with areas of the body and also psychological traits. It is also believed that these centers respond to a *sound* vibration in a therapeutic manner. In western medicine "ultra sound" is used in a variety of ways to help with health conditions. Also *color* is used with the chakras when meditating.

These colors follow the spectrum of the rainbow as you move up the spine. Working with Kundalini energy is said to affect your consciousness and your attitudes, motives, your mental state and your relationships.

See Fig. 5.3 for a diagram and basic information about this theory. Whole books are written on this aspect of yoga. For more information refer to the resources section. It is recommended that this aspect of yoga is best practiced under guidance of a teacher.

Flotation Tanks

"The water had a pleasant viscosity. I felt like a chunk of Dole pineapple in a dish of slowly congealing Jell-O"
... Marc Barasch, *Editorial New Age Journal.* May '84.

This form of relaxation has its origins in the early 1970's when John Lilly M.D., a neuroscientist who had become famous working with the communications skills of dolphins, set up a tank of water at the National Institute of Mental Heallth. The tank is designed so there is no sound or light and you are floating in about 10 inches of water that has 500-800 lbs. of epsom salt dissolved in water at 93.5 degrees. In this state of " sensory deprivation " the physical body can become totally relaxed once you learn to trust the buoyancy of the water. Then your mind can begin to relax and do interesting things. Some people have described their experience as "events" that flash on a "television screen" such as ideas, emotions, childhood memories, images that come and go. The sound of your own breathing and stomach gurgles is amazingly loud at the beginning but as you calm down those sounds also become quieter. The time, usually an hour goes by quickly. When the sound of the New Age music coming out the speakers in the tank signals the end of your session you are amazed and don't want to leave.

So what are the benefits? You will have the feeling of being relaxed, recharged and more alert to all the sensory input in the world- sound, sense of touch and sight. Scientists such as Peter Suedfield of U. of British Columbia and Thomas

Fine of Medical College of Ohio have found that there is an enhancement of learning, IQ scores, visual concentration, recall and perceptual motor tasks. Physically it has been found that endorphins are released and there is also a lowering of blood pressure and the stress-related biochemicals in the blood of those with hypertension.(high blood pressure)

The tanks are now being used by athletes (Philadelphia Phillies won the world series immediately after starting to use the tanks and the Philadelphia Eagles won the Super Bowl); by students to help enhance their learning of chemistry, languages etc; by physicians who recommend it to lower blood pressure, speed healing of broken bones, enhance recovery from heart surgery; by psychiatrists to help patients relieve phobias, depression, anxiety and stress; by creative artists, writers and musicians who use it to tap into their creativity.

Float tanks are one invention of our technological society that allows us to enter a site of tranquility and peace and to allow a renewal of our body and spirit if desired.(See Fig. 5.4) Following are some tips for enjoying and benefitting from your "float".

Before:
   Eat lightly before floating
   Do not shave body hair that day to
      prevent any knicks which the salt
      could irritate.
   Shower before entering the tank
   Put vaseline on any skin abrasions to
      keep salt out
   Put ear plugs in your ears
   You may want to wear a swim or
      shower cap
   Place your towel where you can easily
      find it with your eyes closed
In Tank:
   Locate and practice opening the door
      before lying back in the water.
    Take deep breaths while in the tank
   Find the sides so you know the space
      of your environment in the tank
   Experiment with how you place your
      hands-out to the side, behind neck,
      folded on chest or stomach. Move
      them slowly so you don't drip the
      salt water on your face.
   Allow yourself to relax and don't hold
      your head up
   ENJOY!!!!

Figure 5.3. *Chakra System*

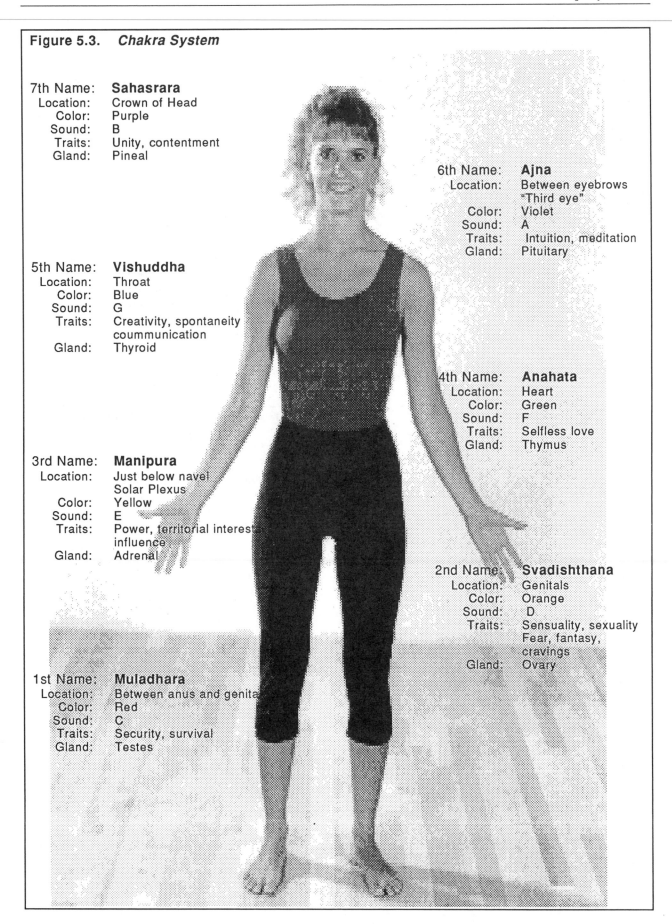

7th Name: **Sahasrara**
Location: Crown of Head
Color: Purple
Sound: B
Traits: Unity, contentment
Gland: Pineal

6th Name: **Ajna**
Location: Between eyebrows
"Third eye"
Color: Violet
Sound: A
Traits: Intuition, meditation
Gland: Pituitary

5th Name: **Vishuddha**
Location: Throat
Color: Blue
Sound: G
Traits: Creativity, spontaneity
coummunication
Gland: Thyroid

4th Name: **Anahata**
Location: Heart
Color: Green
Sound: F
Traits: Selfless love
Gland: Thymus

3rd Name: **Manipura**
Location: Just below navel
Solar Plexus
Color: Yellow
Sound: E
Traits: Power, territorial interest
influence
Gland: Adrenal

2nd Name: **Svadishthana**
Location: Genitals
Color: Orange
Sound: D
Traits: Sensuality, sexuality
Fear, fantasy,
cravings
Gland: Ovary

1st Name: **Muladhara**
Location: Between anus and genitals
Color: Red
Sound: C
Traits: Security, survival
Gland: Testes

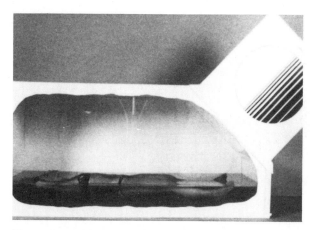

Figure 5.4.   *Flotation Tank*

After:
Take several deep breaths to start to
energize your body
Hold head tilted back when you first
sit up to keep the salty hair
dripping down your back and not
your face
Don't open your eyes until you have a
towel to wipe around hair and face
Shower and shampoo thoroughly
Have a tablet and a pen to take notes
about your experience
Do not plan a day full of activities
following your float

Laughter

We all enjoy a good laugh and the
cleansing and exhausted feeling we have following a bout of the giggles. And now researchers
have discovered just how good laughter really is.
In the following Table 5.3 there is a list of the
body's responses to laughter. We began to take
note of these benefits when Norman Cousins wrote
a book, *Anatomy of an Illness,* in 1979 that was a
chronicle of his bout with a disease of the
connective tissue. He watched old "slapstick
movies" and discovered that "ten minutes of
genuine belly laughter provided at least two hours
of pain free sleep without medication".

I imagine you are wondering how laughter
fits into a yoga class. The routine (Fig. 5.5)
following was developed by a yoga teacher from
India, Swami Dev Murti and was taught to the
English in the 1960's. This routine incorporates
laughter at step 9a and 9b. The whole routine is

a very enjoyable workout, especially for the
back which will be discussed in Unit 7. The
International Yoga Centre in Kent, which was
established by Swami Dev Murti is a delightful
place to stay and to enjoy this style of doing yoga.
Refer to the Resource section for the address of
this center.

Following are some suggestions on how
to add humor and laughter to your daily life.

- Surround your self with people who
  are fun and who will make you laugh
- Look for humor around you
- Laugh at your self
- Have cartoons and funny quotes handy
  so you can see them and laugh
- Do the laughter step 9a and 9b when
  you need a good laugh
- Watch a funny movie when you are
  not feeling well

**Table 5.3.   *Body's Response to
Laughter***

Heart
Doubles the rate for 3-5 minutes in only 20
seconds. Pumps greater amount of blood.
Blood pressure rises temporarily.

Lungs
Ventilation is enhanced as you expel more
of the residual air that stays in lungs between
a normal breath. This allows more oxygen
rich air to be inhaled and you get rid of a
greater amount of carbon dioxide.

Endocrine Glands
ADRENALINE is released and triggers the
pituitary gland to release ACTH (adrenocor-
ticotropic hormone) which stimulates the
kidneys to secrete CORTISOL. The bodys
natural painkiller, ENDORPHIN is then
released. Body produces more immune cells.

Muscular/ Skeletal System
Muscles of scalp, face, neck, shoulders,
chest and abdomen get a workout. Following
laughter there is a reduction of muscle
tension. Arms and legs also can get
involved.

Metabolism
is accelerated and it is estimated that you
burn 78 times as many calories as you do
when you are at rest. This is known as "Inner
Jogging".

Figure 5.5. *Crocodile Routine*

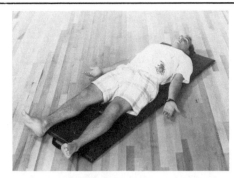

Figure 5.5A.
Basic body position

BASIC BODY POSITION: (Fig. 5.5a) Lie on the back with legs straight and feet together. Arms stretched out sideways level with the shoulders and palms up. Inhale- Push breath down to abdominal cavity. Twist turning the head to the right and the body to the left Slowly roll from side to side as long as breath can be held. Exhale and follow with the -

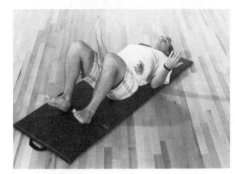

Figure 5.5B.
Fish relaxation

FISH RELAXATION: (Fig. 5.5b) Arms down by sides, bend knees and elbows slightly as inhale and let them drop and flog as exhale. Do 3 times.

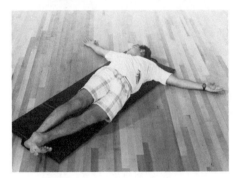

Figure 5.5C.
Foot over ankle

1. Right foot crosses over the left. Keep shoulders on floor on all of the twists.
   FISH RELAXATION

2. Left foot over the right ankle. Twist (Fig. 5.5c)
   FISH RELAXATION

3. Right heel between big toe and next toe of left foot. Twist (Fig. 5.5d)
   FISH RELAXATION

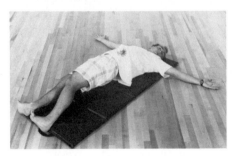

Figure 5.5D.
Heal between big toe and second toe

4. Left heel between big toe and next toe of right foot. Twist
   FISH RELAXATION

5. Bend right knee and place the outside of the right ankle on top (Fig. 5.5e) of the left knee and twist keeping shoulders on the floor.
   FISH RELAXATION

6. Bend left knee and place the outside of the left ankle on top of the right knee and twist keeping shoulders on the floor.
   FISH RELAXATION

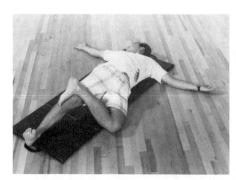

Figure 5.5E.
Ankle on top of knee of other leg

(continued)

Figure 5.5.   *Crocodile Routine*

7.   a. Bend knees, place feet flat and as close to buttocks as possible. Separate feet and knees so that when twisting the right knee touches the floor next to the left heel and vice versa. (Fig. 5.5f) FISH RELAXATION

b. Feet and knees together when twisting this time. The top foot rests on the side of the bottom foot. (Fig. 5.5g)

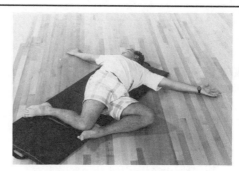

Figure 5.5F.
Knees bent and legs apart

8.   a. Knees to chest and clasp hands behind knees and then roll from side to side with the head going opposite of the knees. (Fig. 5.5h) FISH RELAXATION

b. Knees to chest and roll back onto shoulders and up to a sitting position. FISH RELAXATION

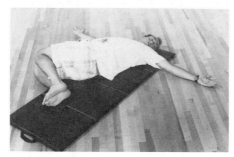

Figure 5.5G.
Knees bent and legs together

9.   a. Basic position but you add a cycling movement with the arms and legs as you laugh loudly on each vowel: HA, HE, HI, HO, HU. Take a new breath for each vowel and laugh until all the air has been expired. (Fig. 5.5i) FISH RELAXATION

b. With the body lying in basic position now laugh with the mouth closed so the air comes out through the nose only. FISH RELAXATION

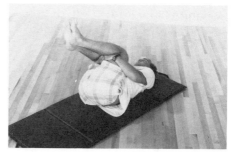

Figure 5.5H.
Knees to chest and rolling

10.   In basic position link the fingers and turn hands so palms are toward the feet. Inhale and slowly with tension on the arms move the hands toward the chest skimming the body surface until you need to exhale. Repeat 2 more times. (Fig. 5.5j) FISH RELAXATION.

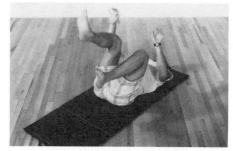

Figure 5.5I.
Cycling with arms and legs and laughing

11.   Arms over head with hands linked, roll several times to right and left. FISH RELAXATION

12.   Sitting up with legs crossed do shoulder rolls:
a.   Both forward and both back
b.   Right forward and left back
c.   Left forward and right back
d.   Both up and both down
e.   One up and one down.
        FISH RELAXATION

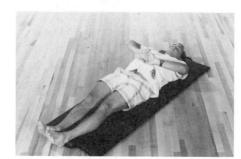

Figure 5.5J.
Hands linked

13.   Deep Relaxation.

SUMMARY

Stress is a part of our lives and the best way to deal with it is to 1)recognize its presence 2) do one or more of the activities suggested in this unit to help alleviate it. Also try some of the following tips to help you deal with stress.

- Slow down and admire nature and the change of seasons.
- Do one thing at a time
- Give yourself time to finish a task
- Sometimes slow down your speaking, eating and walking.
- Take your watch off on the weekends
- Take time each day for some form of relaxing:float tank, listening to music, meditating.

- DON'T feel guilty about relaxing - you deserve it
- Do something for someone else who is "stressed out" and you both will   benefit
- Listen to your body and know when you are pushing too hard
- Try to get enough sleep and follow good eating habits
- Remember how YOU react to stress is under your control!

RESOURCES

Physical Activity and Relaxation

Ardell, Donald, *High Level Wellness,* Bantam, 1979.

Benson, Herbert and Miriam Z Klipper. *The Relaxation Response.* New York, NY: Avon Books, 1979.

_____. "Beyond Relaxation- The Renewable Mind," *American Health-Fitness of Body and Mind.* Sept.1987, p 76-83.

Borysenko, Joan. *Minding the Mody, Mending the Mind.* New York, NY.: Bantam, 1987.

_____. "Love is the Healer", *Yoga Journal,* May/June 1990. P. 45-49,94, 98.

_____. *Guilt is the Teacher, Love is the Lesson.* New York, NY.: Warner, 1990.

Crooks, Cheryl. "Can a Mineral Mitigate Stress?" *American Health-Fitness of Body and Mind.* June, 1985, p. 112.

Goleman, Daniel, and Tara Bennett Goleman. *American Health's Relaxed Body Book.* New York: Doubleday. 1986.

_____. "Moving Toward Mindfullness," *American Health-Fitness of Body and Mind,* March 1987, p. 80-88.

Ornstein, Robert Ph.d, and David Sobel M.D. *Healthy Pleasures.*   Reading, MA: Addison-Wesley Publishing Co. Inc. 1989.

Pelletier, Kenneth R., *Mind as Healer, Mind as Slayer: A Holistic Approach to Preventing Stress Disorders.* New York: Dell, 1977.

Selye, Hans. *Stress Without Distress.* New York. Signet, 1974.

Siegel, Bernie S. M.D. *Love, Medicine and Miracles.*   New York, NY: Harper and Row,Publishers.

_____. *Peace, Love and Healing.* New York, NY: Harper and Row, Publishers. 1989.

Tubesing, Donald. *Kicking the Stress Habit.* Duluth, MN: Whole Person Associates,1982

Pranayama

Iyengar, B.K.S. *Light on Pranayama.* New York, Crossroad Publishing Co., 1981.

 Swami Rama, Rudolph Ballentine, M.D., and Alan Hymes, M.D. *Science of the Breath.* Honesdale, PA, Himalayan Publishers.

Meditation

Ballentine, Rudolph, M.D. *The Theory and Practice of Meditation,* Honesdale, PA, Himalayan Publishers

Christensen, Alice. *The American Yoga Association Beginner's Manual,* New York, Simon & Schuster, Inc. A Fireside Book. 1987.

Biofeedback

The Biofeedback Society of America, 4301 Owens Street, Wheat Ridge, CO 80033, (303)422-8436 Maintains a network of State societies.

The Biofeedback Certification Institute of America, 4301, Owens Street, Wheat Ridge,CO 80033 (303)420-2902
     Provides national certification.
For inexpensive temperature feedback devices:
     Echo, Inc. P.O.Bos 87, Springfield, OH 45501, (513) 322-4972
     Bio-temp Products, Inc. 1950 W. 886th St., Indianapolis, IN 46260, (317)87-9888
     HIMALAYAN INSTITUTE, RR1, Honesdale, PA 18431. 1-800-444-5772

Music
Articles
Halpern, Steve Ph.D., "Musical Meditation",*The 1989 Guide to New Age Living*, p. 62-64.
"Body and Soul Music", *American Health-Fitness ofBody and Mind*, June, 1985, p.66-67.
"Soul Music", *New Age Journal,* April 1987, p. 58-63.

Catalogs
Institute for Music, Health and Education. Director; Don G. Campbell, P.O Box 1244, Boulder, CO 80306.
Heartbeats,from Backroads Distributors, 417 Tamal Plaza, Corte Madera, CA 94925, 1-800-825-4848
Heartsong Review, PO Box 1084, Cottage Grove OR 97424. This is a published twice a year as a resource guide
     for new age music as well as a catalog.
Two-year subscription- $10.00. One-year is $6.00.

Audio Tapes
Campbell, Don. "Angels", "Crystal Rainbows", "Crystal Meditations", "Cosmic Classics".
Enya. "Watermark", and "Enya"
Halpern, Steve. "Dawn". "Spectrum Suite","Crystal Suite", "Gaia's Groove"
_____ and Georgia Kelly, "Ancient Echos"
Rowland, Mike. "The Fairy Ring", "Solace", "Titania", and "Silver Wings".
Solitude Series. Nature Soundtracks- swamps, lakes, oceans, .
Environments Series. Oceans, meadows, forests, thunderstorm, sailboat and ocean
Horn, Paul. "Inside the Pyramids", "Inside the Taj Mahal", "Peace Album"- Christmas
Vollenweider, Andreas. "Caverna Magica", "Behind the Garden...", "Dancing With the Lion", "Down to the
     Moon"

Imagery
Publications
Advances, Journal of the Institute for the Advancement of Health, 16 East 53rd Street, New York, N.Y. 10022
Gawain, Shakti. *Creative Visualization.* New York. Bantam Books,1978.
Institute of Noetic Sciences; P.O. Box 909, Sausalito, CA 94966-0909; (415) 331-5650
Marrone, Robert. *Body of Knowledge: An Introduction to Body/Mind Psychology,* Albany, N.Y. State Univer-
     sity of New York Press. 1990.
Miller, D. Patrick. "Where Scientists and Mystics Meet," *Yoga Journal,* September/October, 1989. p.63-66.
Brain Mind Bulletin. Editor/publisher Marilyn Ferguson, Interface Press, Box 2211, 4717 N. Figueroa St., Los
     Angeles CA 90042.

Video Tapes
Halpern, Steven. "Summer Wind" 35 minutes.
Halpern, Steven, and other musicians. "Natural Light: Windance". 30 minutes

Floating
Hutchison, Michael. "Exploring the Inner Sea",*New Age Journal,* May, 1984. p. 37-43.
_____. *The Book of Floating.* William Morrow and Company. 1984.

Chakras
Audio Tape
Grof, Christina, *"Kundalina"* .

Video Tape
MacLaine, Shirley. "Inner Workout"

Books
"Seven Levels of Consciousness", *Psychology Today,* December 1975.
Iyengar, B.K.S. *Light on Yoga,* New York, Schocken Books, 1965.
Smith,   and Linda Boudreau -Smith. *Yoga for a New Age.*

Laughter
Cousins,Norman. *Anatomy of an Illness.*   New York.   W.W. Norton & Co., 1979.
Peter, Lawrence J.   *The Laughter Prescription.* Ballantine, 1982.
International Yoga Centre, "Highfield" , Lenham, Nr. Maidstone, Kent ME172EX England. Telephone: Lenham 431
   (858431)

The Basic Four, Revisited

The Basic Four you learned in third grade never looked like this! First, we've divvied up each group into "Anytime," "Sometimes," and "Seldom" categories, according to fat, cholesterol, salt, and/or sugar levels. Next we've upped the number of servings of "Grains" to between 6 and 11 (9 on average), and increased "Fruits & Vegetables" to between 5 and 9 (7 on average).

Wondering if you'll have time to do anything but eat bread and carrots all day? Relax. The servings are quite small (1 slice of bread, 1 piece of fruit, or $^1/_2$ cup of rice, pasta, or vegetables, for example).

The chart works best if you compare foods within groups (whole milk vs. skim), not between groups (rice vs. hot dogs).

		Anytime	Sometimes	Seldom
GRAIN GROUP *(6-11 servings a day)* **9**		Whole-grain bread*, rolls*, bagels* Whole-grain crackers* [3], tortillas* Brown rice* Bulgur Whole-grain breakfast cereal* Pasta*	Muffins* [6] Waffles, pancakes* [3] Heavily-sweetened cereals [6] Granola cereals	Croissants [3] Doughnuts [1,6] Danish [6] Bread stuffing from mix [1,3]
FRUIT & VEGETABLE GROUP *(5-9 servings a day)* **7**		All fruits and vegetables (except those at right) Applesauce, unsweetened Potatoes, white or sweet	Avocado [2], guacamole [2] Dried fruit Canned fruit [6] Fruit juice Vegetables, canned with salt [3] French fries, fried in vegetable oil [2]	Coconut [1] Pickles [3] Scalloped or au gratin potatoes [1,3] French fries, fried in beef fat [1] (McDonald's, Burger King, Wendy's)
MILK GROUP *(Children: 3-4 servings a day. Adults: 2 servings a day)* **2**		1% lowfat cottage cheese [3] Dry-curd cottage cheese Skim milk 1% lowfat milk Nonfat yogurt	2% lowfat or regular cottage cheese [3] Reduced-fat or part-skim cheeses [3] 2% lowfat milk Lowfat yogurt, plain or fruit [6] Ice milk [6] Frozen nonfat or lowfat yogurt [6]	Hard cheeses (like cheddar) [1,3] Processed cheeses [1,3] Whole milk [1] Whole-milk yogurt [1] Ice cream [1,6]
FISH, POULTRY, MEAT, EGGS, BEANS, & NUTS GROUP *(2 servings a day)* **2**	**Fish** *(5-oz., roasted)*	All finfish [5] Salmon, canned [3,5] Sardines, in fish oil [3,5] Tuna, water-pack [3] Shellfish, except shrimp	Fried fish [2] Sardines, in vegetable oil [3] Tuna, oil-pack Shrimp [4]	
	Poultry *(4-oz., roasted)*	Chicken breast (without skin) Turkey breast, drumstick, thigh Ground turkey (without skin)	Chicken breast (with skin) Chicken drumstick, thigh Fried chicken, except thigh [2] Ground turkey (with skin)	Fried chicken thigh [2] or wing [2] Chicken hot dog [3]
	Red Meats *(3-oz., trimmed and roasted)*	Pork tenderloin	Round steak, sirloin steak Lean ham [3] Pork or lamb loin chop Leg of lamb, veal sirloin Veal loin or rib chop	Chuck blade[1], rib roast [1] Extra-lean or lean ground beef [1] Pork or lamb[1] rib chop, bacon Bologna [1,3], salami [1,3], Hot dog [1,3] Any untrimmed red meat [1]
	Eggs	Egg white		Whole egg or yolk [4]
	Beans, Peas, & Nuts	Beans, peas, lentils	Tofu [2], peanut butter[2], nuts[2]	

* *refined-grain versions have less fiber, vitamins, and minerals.*
[1] *high in saturated fat*   [2] *high in unsaturated fat*   [3] *may be high in salt or sodium*   [4] *high in cholesterol*   [5] *may be rich in omega-3 fats*   [6] *high in added sugar*

YOGA AND NUTRITION

*"Eat leeks in tide and garlic in May,
and all the year after
Physicians may play."*
. . . Russian Proverb

During the twenty-plus years that I have been a yoga teacher I have observed my students interest in nutrition grow as *they* grew in their yoga practice. It seems that as they became more aware of their body through doing the yoga asanas they gained in respect for their body and its various complex functions one of them being food intake and the effect of appropriate nutrients chemicals, and additives on their body. Over the years the students and I have discussed some of the current trends, fad diets and old established nutrition choices. Since I am not a trained nutritionist I don't pretend to have all the answers but discuss the basics and tell where to go for more information. I see as a benefit of this interest a heightened awareness of the importance of good nutrition habits in their life. This unit is a discussion of what nutrition topics are and have been of interest to my hatha yoga students.

NATIONAL DIETARY GUIDELINES

In 1980, the "Dietary Guidelines for Americans" were established by the United States Department of Agriculture and the United States Department of Health, Education and Welfare now called the Department of Health and Human Services. These were reviewed and in 1985 the following guidelines were agreed upon:

- Eat a variety of foods
- Maintain desirable weight
- Avoid too much fat, saturated fat and cholesterol
- Eat foods adequate in starch and fiber
- Avoid too much sugar
- Avoid too much sodium
- If you drink alcohol, do so in moderation

Table 6.1. *Recommendations: Calorie, Fat and Sodium*

	Age	Average Daily Calorie Intake	Maximum Calories	Fat Grams	Milligrams of Sodium
Children	6-11	2000	500		
Females	12-17	1800	450	44	1100 to 3300
	18-44	1600	400		for adults
	45- up	1400	350		(pregnant
					women
Males	12-17	1800	650	67	need
	18-54	2400	600		more-see
	55-up	2000	500		physician)

Table 6.1 can be a helpful reference as it suggests an average daily caloric intake, the maximum advisable calories from fat, and milligrams of sodium for children, adult males and females.

BASIC 4 FOOD GROUPS PLUS WATER

One of the basic nutrition recommendations is to eat a variety of foods so that you are meeting all of your food needs from the four food groups. You can refer to the following Table 6.2 for the recommended daily servings.

The nutritional needs for protein (fish, poultry, meat & legumes) is recommended to be 12% of the total food intake and is needed to build and repair the body. Carbohydrates, found in the beans, grains, nuts, and vegetables should consist of 58% of the total. These foods provide us with our major source of energy along with fat which should be 30% or less of the total daily intake. Fiber, vitamins and minerals are the other necessary ingredients for a healthy diet.

Water is an often neglected ingredient when discussing nutrition. When exercising, the circulation to the muscles increases and sweating will also occur. Thus the need for water is increased, as it will help rid the body of waste. Water also helps relieve constipation. Eight glasses a day are recommended and even more is all right as it can not hurt you. Bottled water is sometimes necessary when the local water source is known to be impure but watch the sodium content. It should be less than 60 mg per liter.

Table 6.2. *Recommended Daily Nutrition Needs for Adults*	
Beans, Grains, Nuts	- 4 servings daily
Vegetables and Fruits	- 4 servings daily
Milk, Cheese, Yogurt	- 2 servings daily
Fish, Poultry, Meat Legumes	- 2 servings daily

CENTER FOR SCIENCE IN THE PUBLIC INTEREST

This organization, CSPI, was developed as a consumer group to monitor the food industry and also makes recommendations to protect the health of the consumer. They publish a newsletter "Nutrition Action Healthletter", have published books and have also developed posters that have information about salt, sugar, fat and chemical content in food. There is also a chart (Table 6.3 The Basic Four Revisited) that categorizes the foods by the four food groups, listing those most nutritious and identifying what the nutritional shortcoming is.

Michael Jacobson, the director of CSPI since its conception in the early 1970's, has been a guest on many talk shows and on national news sharing nutrition information with the consumer. One of this group's most valuable contributions has been the demand for and the development of food labeling. Learn to read labels so you know what you are getting in the way of hidden fat, sugar, salt and chemicals. When possible make choices that supply your body with more nutritional benefits.

SUPPLEMENTS TO FOOD INTAKE

Commercial Diet Centers and Eating Plans

These programs may serve a purpose for those who are extremely obese and who under a physicians supervision are using these expensive programs to lose weight and change their eating habits. But for those who are slightly over weight or are of a normal weight they are not recommended.

Vitamins and Mineral Supplements

Professional nutritionsts state that if you are eating from the Basic 4 Food Groups the recommended daily servings for you it is not necessary to take vitamin and minerals in a tablet or pill form. But many people, depending on their

Table 6.3. *Basic Four Revisited*

The Basic Four, Revisited

The Basic Four you learned in third grade never looked like this! First, we've divvied up each group into "Anytime," "Sometimes," and "Seldom" categories, according to fat, cholesterol, salt, and/or sugar levels. Next we've upped the number of servings of "Grains" to between 6 and 11 (9 on average), and increased "Fruits & Vegetables" to between 5 and 9 (7 on average).

Wondering if you'll have time to do anything but eat bread and carrots all day? Relax. The servings are quite small (1 slice of bread, 1 piece of fruit, or ¹/₂ cup of rice, pasta, or vegetables, for example).

The chart works best if you compare foods within groups (whole milk vs. skim), not between groups (rice vs. hot dogs).

		Anytime	Sometimes	Seldom
GRAIN GROUP *(6-11 servings a day)* **9**		Whole-grain bread*, rolls*, bagels* Whole-grain crackers* [3], tortillas* Brown rice* Bulgur Whole-grain breakfast cereal* Pasta*	Muffins* [6] Waffles, pancakes* [3] Heavily-sweetened cereals [6] Granola cereals	Croissants [3] Doughnuts [1,6] Danish [6] Bread stuffing from mix [1,3]

FRUIT & VEGETABLE GROUP *(5-9 servings a day)* **7**		All fruits and vegetables
		   (except those at right)
		 Applesauce, unsweetened
		 Potatoes, white or sweet
			Avocado [2], guacamole [2]
			 Dried fruit
			 Canned fruit [6]
			 Fruit juice
			 Vegetables, canned with salt [3]
			 French fries, fried in vegetable oil [2]
				Coconut [1]
				 Pickles [3]
				 Scalloped or au gratin potatoes [1,3]
				 French fries, fried in beef fat [1]
				   (McDonald's, Burger King,
				   Wendy's)

MILK GROUP *(Children: 3-4 servings a day. Adults: 2 servings a day)* **2**		1% lowfat cottage cheese [3] Dry-curd cottage cheese Skim milk 1% lowfat milk Nonfat yogurt	2% lowfat or regular cottage cheese [3] Reduced-fat or part-skim cheeses [3] 2% lowfat milk Lowfat yogurt, plain or fruit [6] Ice milk [6] Frozen nonfat or lowfat yogurt [6]	Hard cheeses (like cheddar) [1,3] Processed cheeses [1,3] Whole milk [1] Whole-milk yogurt [1] Ice cream [1,6]
FISH, POULTRY, MEAT, EGGS, BEANS, & NUTS GROUP *(2 servings a day)* **2**	**Fish** *(5-oz., roasted)*	All finfish [5] Salmon, canned [3,5] Sardines, in fish oil [3,5] Tuna, water-pack [3] Shellfish, except shrimp	Fried fish [2] Sardines, in vegetable oil [3] Tuna, oil-pack Shrimp [4]	
	Poultry *(4-oz., roasted)*	Chicken breast (without skin) Turkey breast, drumstick, thigh Ground turkey (without skin)	Chicken breast (with skin) Chicken drumstick, thigh Fried chicken, except thigh [2] Ground turkey (with skin)	Fried chicken thigh [2] or wing [2] Chicken hot dog [3]
	Red Meats *(3-oz., trimmed and roasted)*	Pork tenderloin	Round steak, sirloin steak Lean ham [3] Pork or lamb loin chop Leg of lamb, veal sirloin Veal loin or rib chop	Chuck blade [1], rib roast [1] Extra-lean or lean ground beef [1] Pork or lamb [1] rib chop, bacon Bologna [1,3], salami [1,3], Hot dog [1,3] Any untrimmed red meat [1]
	Eggs	Egg white		Whole egg or yolk [4]
	Beans, Peas, & Nuts	Beans, peas, lentils	Tofu [2], peanut butter [2], nuts [2]	

* refined-grain versions have less fiber, vitamins, and minerals.
[1] high in saturated fat   [2] high in unsaturated fat   [3] may be high in salt or sodium   [4] high in cholesterol   [5] may be rich in omega-3 fats   [6] high in added sugar

work schedule, budget, where they are living, (residence hall, sharing an apartment, or living with parents) do not always meet those daily recommendations. So examine your lifestyle and your present eating habits to see what **YOU** are doing. You don't want to waste your money on "expensive urine", as nutritionists suggest can happen with the water soluble vitamins (C and B complex). If more of the fat soluble vitamins (A, D, E and K) are taken into the body than you use they will be stored and can cause health problems. Check with a physician and nutritionist about this concern. Vitamins and minerals such as calcium, are important to the body as they regulate various body processes and help maintain body tissue and bone. Refer to the Nutrition Action Healthletter listed at the end of this unit for more information about the use of supplements.

Garlic

"But for its odour -
garlic would be costlier than gold".
...Charak- father of Hindu medicine.

This pleasant but sometimes potent seasoning ingredient has been in the news concerning its potential to help lower cholesterol, increase the bloods ability to clot, function as a natural antibiotic and to strengthen the immune system. Research has been conducted in Europe, Japan and India for years on the effects of garlic on overall health. The history of garlic goes back 5,000 years where it is mentioned in Sanskrit manuscripts from India. It was also known to be used in China 3,000 years ago and in Egypt in 3750 B.C. when the pyramids were being built. It is also mentioned in the Hebrew book, the Talmud, where it states that taking garlic will help destroy "parasites". The Old Testament states that when journeying through the desert, sufficient rations of garlic went along. One of the most famous garlic stories is from the Middle Ages when the bubonic plague was on the rampage in Europe. It is reported that those who ate garlic in their diet survived at a ratio of three to one over non-garlic eaters.

This brings us to the question-What are the properties in garlic which brings about these effects on the body? The following have been identified and researched.

Allicin - has anti-inflammatory and anti-bacterial effect

Allithiamine (Vitamin B1) - helps prevent nervous and skin ailments

Selenium - helps prevent the build up of fatty placque in the blood vessels

Diallyldisulphide Oxide - this ingredient is what results when allicin is converted in the body and this is what is believed to lower the cholesterol and the lipids (fat substances) in the blood

Amino Acids - cystine and methionine which promote cellular growth and healing

Thiamine - helps with metabolism of carbohydrates and also coping with stress

Garlic has been used as a major ingredient in the cuisine of India, China and the Mediterranean area. When I stayed at a yoga center in England I was told to eat two to three fresh whole cloves of garlic with every meal as it was good for my circulation. To help overcome the after effects of eating raw garlic you can try one of the following remedies.

- Rinse mouth with 1/2 water and 1/2 lemon juice
- Chew on dill, fennel or anise seed
- Chew on roasted coffee ground and then spit out
- Eat a fresh apple
- Chew a slice of cinnamon or a whole clove
- Chew pieces of orange peel

Garlic is easy to grow and inexpensive to purchase. It is easy to develop the habit of cooking with garlic to enhance naturally your favorite recipes and remember this New York Yiddish saying- "Three nickles will get you on the subway but garlic will get you a seat."

THREE APPROACHES TO EATING

Vegetarianism

Some people think that to properly "do yoga" you have to be a vegetarian or have no red meat in your diet. This is not true. Yoga did develop in India, where people do not eat meat for a variety of reasons ranging from religion, dietary choices to economical and just plain personal choice. There are several categories of a vegetarian diet.

Traditional vegetarians: those whose eating habits have existed over generations due to a cultural belief and or lifestyle

Total "vegans": no animal products at all are eaten

Lacto-vegetarians: dairy products are eaten

Lacto-ovo vegetarians: dairy products and eggs are eaten

Semi-vegetarians: consume some groups of animal foods (possibly no red meat but fish and chicken might be eaten

New vegetarians: developed after the 1960's, eat some form of a vegetarian diet along with foods that are considered to be less processed and more natural or organic.

Many of the vegetarian diets are "millenia old and have stood the test of time with respect to the propagation of the species" as stated in the Journal of American Dietetics Association position paper on vegetarianism. (1980- Vo. 77 p. 61-69)

A vegetarian diet is usually low in saturated fat and high in dietary fiber which are highly recommended eating habits. Research studies done on Seventh-Day Adventisits, who practice lacto-ovo and/or vegan eating habits, have shown that they have a lower mortality rate from coronary heart disease and cancer than the rest of our American population. (see resources list at end of unit)

There are several factors to consider when planning a vegetarian type diet.

1. Select from a variety of the Basic 4 food group substituting the peas, beans and nuts for the meat group.
2. Monitor the intake of the dairy group as you many need to increase the servings here.
3. Reduce (or eliminate) the empty calorie foods in your diet. (those that are high in calories and low in nutrients).
4. Increase the intake of complex carbohydrates (whole grain breads and cereals) to meet your energy requirements.
5. Combine: beans and wheat; beans and rice; lentils and rice; to get the amino

acids from the protein that is necessary.
6. If you are not consuming animal dairy products:
   a. drink fortified soybean milk
   b. provide Vitamin D as a supplement (check with physician)
   c. provide Vitamin B 12 as a supplement or eat foods high in B 12 (cereals, eggs, soybean products made to resemble meat - read labels)

If you are curious about what a day's menu based on a vegetarian diet is like refer to Table 6.4 for a sample menu for a lacto-ovo vegetarian diet.

Anti-Cancer Diet

Research in epidemiology in the last ten years has made some connections between dietary habits, dietary intake and cancer. It has been discovered that the following nutrients may have a positive impact on lowering the risk of cancer:

Cruciferous vegetables - (broccoli, brussel sprouts, cabbage, cauliflower, bok choy, collord greens, kale, kohlrabi, mustard and turnip greens, rutabagas and turnips)

Beta carotene - converted to Vitamin A in the body. (carrots, apricots, cantaloupe, papayas, nectarines, watermelon, broccoli, sweet potatoes, winter squash and all dark leafy vegetables.)

Vitamin C - helps with cellular strengthening (primarialy citrus)

Vitamin E - (peppers, spinach, carrots, broccoli, rice, wheat and oats, yeast and vegetable oils, and liver),

Fiber - (whole grains and fresh fruits and vegetables)

The American Institute for Cancer Reserch has a newsletter and numerous pamphlets that are helpful when learning how to lower cancer risk. They have outlined recommendations which are similar to the guidelines from the United States Government and the Center for Science in the Public Interest. These AICR suggestions resulted from the work of nutritionist Jerry Rivers Ph D. and Karen Collins, M.S., R. D.

Table 6.4   *Vegetarian Eating Plan*

Sample Menus for Lacto-ovovegetarian Diet

Meal and Food Group	Menu 1	Menu 2
Breakfast		
Milk	Milk	Milk
Meat Alternate		Scrambled egg or tofu (soy curd)
Fruit-Vegetable	Orange	Prune juice
Grain	Oatmeal	Shredded wheat
	Date-nut muffin	Wheat soy bread
Others	Butter/margarine	Butter/margarine
	Coffee/hot cereal	Coffee/ hot cereal
	Beverage	Beverage
Lunch		
Milk	Cream Mushroom Soup (made with milk)	Cottage Cheese for Fruit Plate
Meat Alternate	Peanut Butter for Sandwich	Lentil Soup
Fruit-Vegetable	Carrot Sticks	Apricots, Grapefruit
	Banana	Pineapple, Grapes, Lettuce Leaves in Fruit Plate
Grain	Rye Crackers	Whole Wheat Crackers
	Whole Wheat Bread	
Others	Beverage	Salad Dressing
		Beverage
Dinner		
Milk	Yogurt	
Meat Alternate	Baked Beans	Quiche - milk, egg
Fruit-Vegetable	Corn	Broccoli
	Collards	Spinach Salad
	Sliced Tomato Salad	
Grain	Brown Bread	Whole Wheat Roll
Others	Salad Dressing	Salad Dressing
	Butter/ Margarine	Butter/ Margarine
	Tea/ Hot Cereal	Tea/ Hot Cereal
	Beverage	Beverage
Snacks	Cheese	Sunflower Seeds
	Crackers	Apple

Vegetarian Nutrition. National Dairy Council. 1979, Rosemont, IL 60018

1. Reduce the intake of dietary fat- both saturated and unsaturated.
2. Increase the consumption of fruits, vegetables and whole grain cereals.
3. Consume salt-cured, smoked and charcoal-broiled foods only in moderation.
4. Drink alcoholic beverages only in moderation.

You may want to refer to a sample menu from AICR, Table 6.5, which is based upon the above recommendations. The recipe will be in the recipe section.

Longevity Diet

A diet that is "high" in nutrient quality and "low" in calories is recommended by Roy L. Walford, M.D., a professor of Pathology at the University of California at Los Angeles and one of this country's leading researchers in the field of

Table 6.5.   *Anit-Cancer Eating Plan*

Menu Using all Food Groups

Breakfast
1/4 cup Ready-to-Eat Whole Grain Cereal
    1/2 cup Cantaloupe
    1/2 cup Lowfat Milk
1 1/2 cup Skim or Lowfat Milk

Salad Bar Lunch
Salad Bar with Small Wedge Lettuce
    1/2 cup Carrots
    1/4 cup Raw Cauliflower
    1/2 cup Garbanzo or Kidney Beans
    2 Tbsp. Regular Salad Dressing
6 Whole Grain Rye Wafers

Quick-to-Fix Dinner
6 oz. chicken (or Veal)
Piccata (pounded very thin, cooked quickly, and
    flavored with lemon and parsley)
1cup Whole Wheat Noodles
    with 1 1/2 tsp. Margarine
1/4 cup Tomato-Basil Salad

Evening Snack
1 Bran Muffin

---

aging and life extension. He recommends that we "increase the ratio of fish to red meat in the diet, increase vegetable protein in relation to animal protein (this will lower the amount of fat in the diet), increase the amount of complex carbohydrates, cut back sharply on refined sugars, and make sure that copper and chromium intake are not greatly below the Recommended Daily Allowance levels." (Walford, p. 124) He also suggest that you raise your magnesium intake over the current average amount, let the ratio of magnesium/calcium in your diet be 1.1 and increase the intake of gel-forming fibers such as bran. He recommends adequate calcium and lower amounts of fat and sodium to help protect the body from diseases. Dr. Walford's book, *The 120-Year Diet* (1986), discusses in great detail the impact of good nutrition practices on the body. It presents 20 days of computer-generated, nutrient dense, low-calorie menus with recipes, as well as a chart of the nutritive values of the best foods. This book is full of sound nutritional advice. (see resources) Following is a sample menu in Table 6.6 and the recipe will be in the recipe section on page78-79.

Table 6.6.   *Longevity Eating Plan*

Day Three

Breakfast

1/4 cup rolled oats	25 gm
1/2 cup wheat bran	20 gm
1 tbsp. yeast	5 gm
1 banana sliced	150 gm
1 glass skim milk	244 gm

Lunch

1/4 pound marinated halibut	100 gm
1/2 cup cabbage (as cole slaw)	50 gm
1 glass skim milk	244 gm

Dinner

Oyster cocktail	
(4 to 8 oysters, depending on size)	100 gm
Pasta Primavera	1 serving
6-8 leaves kale, steamed,	
with sauce of choice	50 gm
1 slice watermelon,	
equivalent of 2 cups, diced	320 gm

Nutritional Information

Total Calories	1,142
% Calories From Fat	11
Total Protein	76 gm
Total Carbohydrates	178 gm
Total Fat	14 gm

% of RDA's

Tryptophan	538
Isoleucine	522
Lysine	742
Valine	506
Methionine, cysteine	455
Threonine	630
Leucine	601
Phenylalanine, tyrosine	599
Vitamin A	256
Vitamin D	150
Vitamin K	674
Vitamin C	511
Vitamin E	73
Riboflavin	116
Vitamin B 6	156
Vitamin B 12	698
Thiamine	165
Niacin	146
Folacin	138
Pantothenic Acid	169
Biotin	74
Calcium	96
Magnesium	115
Copper	227
Zinc	338
Chromium	177
Phosphorus	144
Potassium	208
Iron	102
Manganese	158
Selenium	283

Reprinted with permission of Simon and Schuster, from *The 120 Year Diet* by Roy L. Walford, M.D. © 1986 p.268.

SUMMARY

There is much information in this unit which may have overwhelmed you. To help you sort through all of this I will attempt to pull it all together with some basic suggestions that have appeared throughout and add a few more. First, eating should be pleasurable, but not the central focus of your life. Think of food as providing the fuel, and necessary ingredients to keep your body running for a long and healthy life. Second, remember this basic idea using the yoga approach-Try to eat foods as close to their natural state as your digestion permits. Third, read food labels. Fourth, keep your nutrient and fiber content HIGH. Fifth, keep *low* the fat and fried foods, overprocessed foods, and your total caloric intake (at levels desirable for you). Sixth, DAILY eat from all 4 food groups, some of the anti-cancer foods and a little garlic!

RESOURCES

Books
Brody, Jane. *Jane Brody's Nutrition Book.* New York, N.Y.; W.W. Norton & Co., 1981.
Gilroy, People of. *The Complete Garlic Lovers' Cookbook.* Berkeley. CA Celestial Arts. 1987.
Hausman, Patricia and Judith Benn Hurley. *The Healing Foods,* Emmaus, PA. Rodale Press, 1989.
Lappe, FrancesMoore. *Diet for A Small Planet.* New York: Ballantine Books. 1982.
Madison, Deborah. *The Greens Cook Book*
Robertson, Laurel, et al. *Laurel's Kitchen.*   Nilgiri Press.
Walford, Roy MD. *The 120 Year Diet.* New York, N.Y.; Simon and Schuster, Inc. 1986.

Articles
Hurley, Jayne and Stephen Schmidt. "A Clove a Day?", *Nutrition Action Healthletter.* December, 1989, p. 8-9.
Liebman, Bonnie. "Getting Your Vitamins?" *Nutrition Action Healthletter.* June 1990, p. 1, 5-7.
_____ "Carrots Against Cancer?" *Nutrition Action Healthletter.* December 1988, p. 1, 5-7.
"Making the Most of Fast Food Meals." *American Institute for Cancer Research Newsletter.* Summer 1990.
        p. 6.

Magazine To Subscribe To
American Institute for Cancer Research Newsletter. Publlished by the American Institute for Cancer Research. 1759 R. Street N.W. Washington, D.C. 20009, telephone (202) 328-7744.
Nutrition Action Healthletter. Published by the Center for Science in the Public Interest. 1501 16th St., N.W. Washington, D. C. 20036.
Vegetarian Times. P.O. Box 446 Mt. Morris, IL 61054-9894.

RECIPES

Oat and Wheat Pancakes

You can mix this easy batter up to 18 hours ahead. Refrigerate, then stir before using. 1 1/4 cups oats and 2 cups skim milk- mix and let stand 10 mins. Stir in 1 egg, 1/2 cup all-purpose flour, 1/4 cup toasted wheat germ, 1 Tb. sugar, 1Tb. baking powder, 2 tsp. vegetable oil and 1/2 tsp salt. For each pancake pour a scant 1/4 batter on hot well-greased griddle over medium-low heat. Cook turning once, until well browned on both sides and cooked through. Makes 12 pancakes. *Per pancake; 92 cal, 4 g pro, 14, g car, 2 g fat, 22 mg chol, 201 mg sod.*

Nebraska Bran Muffins

From *Diet for a Small Planet*, Frances Moore Lappe', p. 325, Ballantine Books, New York. 1979.

In a large bowl mix and let stand: 3 cups bran flakes (can substitue part All-Bran cereal) and 1 cup boiling water. Beat in medium bowl 2 eggs, 1 1/4 cup sugar or 1 cup honey, 2 cups buttermilk, 1/2 cup corn or other oil. Add to bran mixture. Sift together 2 cups whole wheat flour, 1/2 cup soy flour, 2 1/2 tsp soda, 1/2 tsp salt and fold into bran. Bake at 370° for 15 minutes in a greased muffin tin. A variation of these muffins was developed for the Nebraska centennial in1966. The addition of the soy is quite fitting and increases the protein content and usability. The batter may be refrigerated in covered jars several weeks. 2 muffins =approximately 6g usable protein, 14-17% of daily protein allowance.

Irish Soda Bread

This bread does not need any time to rise but it should sit about 6 hours after it comes out of the oven before it is sliced. If the crust seems too hard, wrap the baked bread in a damp teal towel and stand upright until it is cool. I like to bake this bread in a cast iron skillet with another skillet or an ovenproof lid to cover. This is more like the way it was originally made in Ireland over a peat fire in a fireplace. Mix 4 cups stone-ground whole-wheat flour, 2 cups white flour, 1 1/2 tsp salt, 1 1/2 tsp baking soda. Make a well in the center and gradually mix in 2 cups buttermilk, sour milk or sweet milk. You may need less, or more liquid-it depends on the absorbent quality of the flour. The dough should be soft and manageable, Knead dough into a ball in the mixing bowl with floured hands. Put in lightly floured skillet and flatten out till touching sides. Make a cross with a floured knife through the center of the bread so it will easily break in quarters when it is baked. Bake at 425° for 25 minutes, reduce the heat to 350 ° and bake a further 15 minutes.

Birkel's Tabouli

Place 1 1/4 cup bulgur in bowl and cover with very hot water and let stand until light and fluffy. Mix 1 cup minced, fresh mint, 2 cups minced parsley, 1 small cucumber seeded and chopped, 4-6 small radishes chopped, 1 small onion chopped or 6 green topped onions, 1/2 green pepper, and 2 chopped tomatoes and add all to bulgur. DRESSING: 3/4 cup lemon juice, 1/4 cup olive oil, 1/2tsp salt, and 1/2 tsp cumin. Chill and serve on lettuce leaf. Will not spoil like a cream type salad. Good for summer picnics. Serves 6-8.

Tomato-Basil Salad (Anti-Cancer)

Slice 4 medium tomatoes, and 1 small red onion thinly; Mix with 1/4 cup fresh basil (or 2 tsp. dried basil. Pour 1/4- 1/3 cup red wine vinegar over the salad and add black pepper to taste. Let marinate at least 1/2 hour, preferably 1-2 hours. Serves 4-5.

Tofu Onion Garlic Dip

Combine all in a blender and mix until smooth: 1 lb. tofu, 1/4 c. oil, 3 tbsp. vinegar, 1 tsp garlic powder (or real garlic minced), 1 medium onion, minced and 1 tbsp soy sauce.(if desired). Serve with crackers or fresh vegetables suce as broccoli, celery, etc.

Tofu Cheesecake

Crust: Preheat oven to 350° In a 9" pie pan, melt 1/2 c. margarine add 1 package graham crackers crushed into fine crumbs. Bake 10 mins. and set aside.

Filling: Combine all in a blender and mix until smooth: 24oz. tofu (or 1 lb tofu and 8 oz. cream cheese), 2 eggs, 2/3 cup honey, (or 1/2 cup sugar), 1 Tbsp vanilla, 2 Tbsp. vegetable oil, 1 Tbsp lemon juice, 1/8 tsp nutmet, 1/4 tsp salt. Pour the filling into the crust and bake at 350 for 40 min (or until golden brown). Top with your favorite fruit or eat plain.

Homemade Lowfat Yogurt

Soften 1/4 tsp gelatine and add boiling water to make 1 cup. Add 1/2 Tbl sugar and cool. Mix 1 1/2 cup instant milk (dry powdered) with 1 1/2 cups water, add 1 small can evaporated milk and 1 more cup of tepid water and the gelatin mixture. Add 1 1/2 TBL of yogurt and stir thoroughly. If you have a yoguty maker fil the jars and let them set for 10 hours. Or pour the mixture into clean glasses or small jars. Put the jars in a large pan of warm water. Cover the jars with clear plastic wrap. Place in a warm oven. Maintain the temperature of water between 100 ° and 120° F. Or set the pan over a pilot light on the stove covered with a towel or blanket. The yogurt will take 3 to 5 hours to thicken and then refrigerate. The yogurt can be lift to sit overnight and then be refrigerated in the morning. Very good and cheap to make. Try it.

Pasta Primavera
(Longevity)- 2 servings

1/4 lb. whole-wheat noodles (fettuccine)130 gm.
1/2 onion, chopped 90 gm.
1 clove elephant garlic, or 4-6 cloves regular garlic, finely chopped 25 gm.
1 tsp. olive oil
4-5 French morel mushrooms, fresh or 20 gms. dried (chopped)
1/2 medium red bell pepper 50 gm.
1 medium tomato 120 gm.
1/2 cup chopped parsley 80 gm.
4 tbsp. finely chopped fresh dill 20 gm.
1/4 to 1/2 cup Enricos spaghetti sauce (or a substitute)
3 tbsp. Salsa
1/2 inch cube parmesan cheese, grated 25 gm.

Place noodles in briskly boiling water for 10 minutes. While they are cooking fry onion and garlic in oil in nonstick skillet until onion is translucent. Add fresh or rehydrated mushrooms and cook for 1 minute then add chopped pepper, tomato, parsley, and dill. Stir completly. Add spaghetti sauce and salsa and simmer 3-5 minutes until parsly is thoroughly cooked. Place noodles on plate, cover with sauce, and sprinkle with parmesan cheese.

Nutritional Information (per serving)

Total calories	358
%calories from fat	15
Total protein	16 gm.
Total carbohydrates	60 gm.
Total fat	6 gm.

% RDAs (per serving)

Tryptophan	117
Isoleucine	103
Lysine	126
Valine	99
Methionine, cysteine	87
Threonine	95
Leucine	118
Phenylalanine, tyrosine	141
Vitamin A	104
Vitamin D	2
Vitamin K	550
Vitamin C	234
Vitamin E	13
Riboflavin	22
Vitamin B_6	21
Vitamin B_{12}	8
Thiamine	35
Niacin	25
Folacin	30
Pontothenic acid	40
Biotin	12
Calcium	22
Magnesium	28
Copper	16
Zinc	18
Chromium	58
Phosphorus	34
Potassium	46
Iron	31
Manganese	18
Selenium	91

YOGA FOR SPECIAL CONDITIONS

May all be happy,
May all be free from disease,
May all look to the good of others,
May none suffer from sorrow.
. . . Anoynomous

Yoga has been recommended as an exercise program for many people who have a limitation of some type. It has also been used as a form of therapy for common problems such as headaches, constipation, back problems or a lack of flexibility. Mr. B.K.S. Iyengar's book *Light on Yoga* has a section where all forms of health conditions are listed with the appropriate yoga asana that can possibly help with the condition. Another good reference for therapeutic hatha yoga for the back has been written by physician, Mary Pullig Schatz.

In this section some of the most common concerns as exhibited by my students will be discussed. What should not be done will be mentioned as well as modifications of the traditional poses when that is feasible. The Asanas that are especially helpful will also be listed. You can refer to the chart, Table 7.1 for a handy reference to locate the poses that should NOT be done or are done with caution.

MENSTRUAL DISORDERS

Judith Lasater, P.T. and Ph.D., recommends for premenstrual syndrome (PMS) that women do the shoulder stand and the forward bending and twisting poses.

Table 7.1.	*Special Conditions and Yoga Asanas*									
Code:	∗ Avoid doing			Δ Do With Caution						
	Breath (Hold)	Shoulder Stand	Dog	Hang HeadStand	Dolphin	Chest Expansion	Bow	Full Locust	Cobra	Plough
Menstrual Cramps		∗		∗						
Pregnant	∗	∗	Δ	∗			∗	∗	∗	∗
High Blood Pressure	∗	Δ		∗	Δ	Δ				∗
Eye Concern	Δ	Δ	Δ	∗	Δ	Δ		Δ		
Neck		Δ		∗				Δ	Δ	∗
Low Back							Δ	Δ	Δ	∗
Scoliosis				Δ						
Overweight		∗		∗				Δ		∗

Precautions

The inverted pose of the shoulder stand, headstand hang and headstand are not to be done DURING the menstrual cycle.

Recommended Asanas for Menstral Disorders

Cat (figure 3.20 on page 24)
Spinal Twist (figure 3.33 on page 37)
Arrow Sit (figure 3.39 on page 42)
Sitting Forward Bend (figure 3.17 on page 21)
Dog (figure 3.21 on page 25)
Back Pushup (figure 3.28 on page 33)
Headstand (figure 3.38 on page 41)*
Shoulder Stand (figure 3.22 on page 26)*
Fish (figure 3.23 on page 28)

* DO NOT do during menstrual cycle.

PREGNANCY

Hatha yoga, in its gentle approach and use of the breath, is an ideal form of exercise during pregnancy. It will improve your circulation and help keep your muscles pliant and can even make the delivery easier. Always remember to do the relaxation daily as this will assist you during delivery. Try to maintain an erect standing posture to protect the muscles of the low back. During pregnancy the breasts become larger to prepare for nursing thus the pectoral muscles underneath the breasts should be strengthened.

Precautions

1. When doing your Pranayama do not hold the breath. Keep the breath flowing in and out.
2. Do NOT do the inverted poses', or headstand hang, headstand or shoulderstand as there is the possibility of placing the fetus next to the top part of the uterus where it may be attached to the placenta. This could place too much pressure at this site.
3. Once the abdomen is becoming large do not do the asanas requiring you to lie on your abdomen. You will know when as it will no longer feel comfortable or "right" for you.

Recommendations

1. Practice the deep breathing daily.
2. In the early stages do the abdominal toning exercises or yoga sitback and up and the single abdominal lift.
3. Elevate your legs by the wall as taught in Unit 3 (figure 3.22a).
4. Check yourself in the mountain pose (figure 3.12) in front of a mirror every week to monitor your postural alignment.
5. Do a standing balance asana daily . As your abdomen increases your sense of balance and center of gravity are changing. Daily practice should help you stay more centered as well as strengthen the feet and legs. Practice by a chair or wall for support.
6. Practice sitting in a squat position. Again use a chair or wall to stabalize yourself if you want. (figure 7.1)
7. Practice sitting in a wide straddle position also. (figure 7.3)
8. Post Pregnancy: When you have approval of your physician begin toning your abdominal muscles. If a cesearean section has been done you will need to be more cautious. The pelvic tilt, cat, and yoga sit back are good ones to begin with as well as the single abdominal lift. You must put effort into strengthening these muscles as soon as you can.
9. Check the resources section for books and videos for yoga during pregnancy and for relaxation music for infants.

Recommended Asanas for Pregnancy

Mountain Pose (figure 3.12 on page 18)
Tree (figure 3.24 on page 29)
Chest Expansion (figure 3.19 on page 23)
Squatting (figure 7.1 on page 81)
Knee Thigh Stretch (figure 7.2 on page 81)
Straddle Sitting (figure 7.3 on page 81)
Cat (figure 7.4 on page 81)
Dog (figure 7.5 on page 81)
Legs Elevated by Wall (figure 3.22a, 7.6 on page 26, 82)
Spinal Twist (figure 7.7 on page 82)

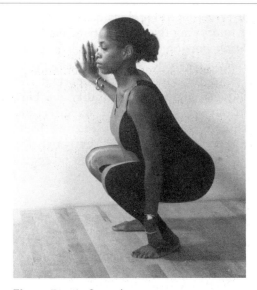

Figure 7.1.   *Squatting*

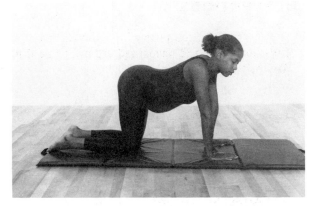

Figure 7.4a.   *Cat*

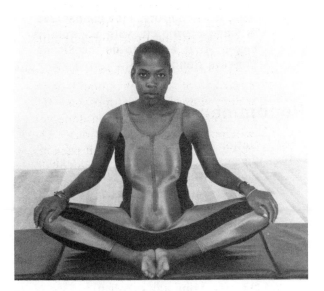

Figure 7.2.   *Knee Thigh Stretch*

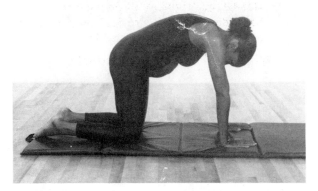

Figure 7.4b.   *Cat*

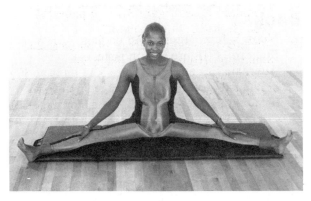

Figure 7.3.   *Straddle Sitting*

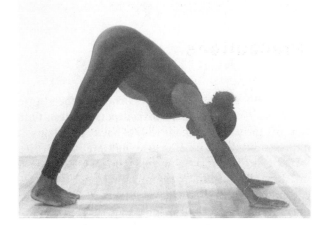

Figure 7.5.   *Dog*

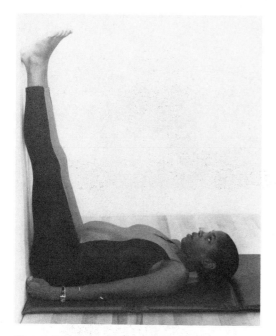

Figure 7.6.   *Legs Elevated by Wall*

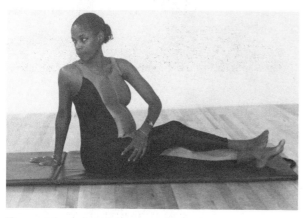

Figure 7.7.   *Spinal Twist*

BACK PROBLEMS

Back ache and pain is probably the single most expensive problem that affects adults. One out of three Americans have back problems - approximately 75 million at some time in their life will be bothered. Each year roughly another 5 million will strain or sprain their back. It is estimated that 83% of the problems are caused by muscular weakness, tension and stress. The lack of flexibility of the back from the head to the toes, weak abdominal muscles, bad posture habits and lack of proper lifting and carrying technique are also causes. This is where yoga comes in. Overall posture is stressed whether in a sitting,

standing or lying position. Yoga asanas are well known for improving the flexibility of the body. The relaxation portion of a yoga class also has beneficial effect on those with back problems.

In yoga the spine is very important. To help maintain strength and flexibility the back needs to be moved gently in all six directions daily - bending forward, gentle arching back, leaning to the right and the left and gently twisting to the right and the left. The routine presented will accomplish this.

Precautions

1. The full locust can aggravate an existing problem in the lumbar area. Do with caution after back has become stronger. Don't lift legs very high.
2. Do not do Standing Forward Bend if there is discomfort in the lumbar area or have a problem with the sciatic nerve. It is better to do the Sitting Forward Bend.

Recommendations

1. Notice how your back feels as you do the poses. Notice if one side is tighter than the other.
2. Do the routine for backs daily.
3. Do some of the preparation poses at the beginning and end of the day.
4. Vary your sleeping posture and don't use a large pillow as it pushes the head forward.
5. Observe your habits when carrying, sitting and standing.

Recommended Asanas for Backs

Moon Salute (figure 3.46 on page 46)
Body rolls (figure 3.3 on page 14)
Alternate Leg stretch (figure 3.11 on page 17)
Pelvic tilt (figure 3.28 on page 33)
Feldenkrais knee overs (figure 3.9 on page 16)
Cobra (figure 3.13 on page 19)
1/2 Locust (figure 3.14 on page 19)
Fetus or Knees to Chest (figure 3.15 or 3.16 on page 20)
Yoga sit back and up (figure 3.32 on page 36)
Abdominal Lift (figure 3.27 on page 32)

The Crocodile Routine, taught by Swami Đev Murti, that is in Unit 5 is most beneficial as the back muscles are freed from some of the effects of gravity. Doing the gentle exercises horizontal means that no vertebrae or muscle is holding up another one and thus the back is allowed to twist more easily. Do this routine daily.

SCOLIOSIS

This is a condition in the spine which allows the vertebrae to curve to the side which affects the rib cage, the shoulder, the hips and a change in the center of gravity. Adolescence is a time when structural scoliosis, which is an unequal growth of the two sides of the vertebrae, develops. Functional scoliosis develops usually from poor posture habits and unbalanced activity such as always carrying your book bag or back pack on the same shoulder. Yoga exercises can help with functional scoliosis and with structural scoliosis if it is identified soon enough.

Precautions

The Headstand should be done with care and supervised by an experienced yoga teacher if you have scoliosis.

Recommendations

1. Take the pressure of off the concave side of the spine. (See Fig. 7.8)
2. Flex the spine in the opposite direction of the concave curve.
3. Twisting the spine can also help relieve the stretch and tension on the convex side. (See Fig. 7.8)
4. Always visualize *extending* the spine upward.
5. Hang from the knees on bar or a jungle gym to allow the back to stretch and relieve the compression between the vertebrae.
6. Practice Pranayama to help keep the thoracic area flexible.
7. See the resource section for articles in the Yoga Journal for those with scioliosis.

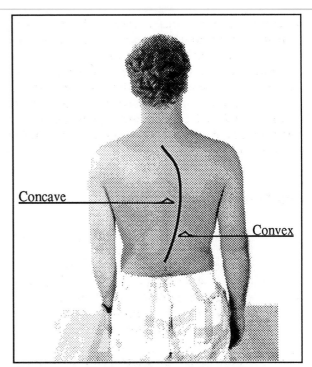

Figure 7.8. *Concave and convex side of spine*

Recommended Asanas for Scoliosis

Downward Facing Dog (figure 3.21 on page 25)

Triangle (figure 3.25 on page 30): Do first on the concave side, repeat to the convex side and a third time on the concave side.

Triangle Twist (figure 3.26 on page 31): Do on concave side as it will then derotate the spine.

Relaxation pose with a conscious effort to line the spine as straight as possible.

NECK INJURY

Many people have injured their neck in a variety of ways. A common injury is a "whiplash" which can leave the muscles of the neck sore and weakened. The alignment of the cervical vertebrae is not always corrected and can lead to tension and muscle fatigue. Yoga poses can assist in strengthening these muscles. You should have permission from your physician to begin exercising. If you have been given a set of exercises to do, share them with your yoga teacher. Precautions to remember: do not do any poses which will hyperextend the neck, like the shoulderstand on a flat surface; when doing the fish which has you lift your head (which weighs 12-15 pounds) you are putting a load on the muscles - DON'T do if it causes pain; DON'T do the headstand hang or the headstand without careful supervision.

Recommendations

1. Always be aware of how you are holding your head over your spine. If you get in the habit of monitoring the head and have it centered over the strong bones of the spine there is a lot less work for the neck muscles to do.
2. Do some gentle stretches and turns frequently during the day.
3. Don't sleep on a large pillow as that pushes your head forward. You can purchase a pillow that is designed to fit the natural curve of the cervical spine.
4. Trade neck massages with friends often.
5. When studying, typing, drawing etc. take frequent breaks to change position and do some of the stretches recommended in the following routine.
6. Keep the head in a straight alignment at all times- for instance keep the chin and not the cheek on the mat when doing the 1/2 locust

Recommended Asanas for Necks

Neck stretches and neck turns (figure 3.1 and 3.2 on page 14)
Chest Expansion (figure 3.19 on page 23)
Head lift and turn; strengthens the front of the neck. (figure 3.8 on page 16)
Fish (figure 3.23 on page 28)
Dog (figure 3.21 on page 25)
Dolphin (figure 3.36 on page 39): Maintain most of the weight with the arms and gradually shift some to the neck being very aware of how the neck feels when you do that. Stop if it hurts.

OVERWEIGHT

When beginning to do yoga people usually develop a greater appreciation for their physical self and thus want to take better care of themself. This can lead to changes in eating (Unit 6) and exercise habits. Hatha yoga in its gentle approach can be done by those who are overweight.

Precautions

Inverted poses should be done with caution:
1. Headstand hang and headstand not at all
2. Shoulder stand by the wall
3. Dolphin for a short time and then repeating 2 times.

ARTHRITIS

Hatha yoga poses are recommended for those with arthritis. The manner in which the asanas are done are very helpful to those with arthritis. Today the Arthritis Foundation and many physicians recognize that exercise help to improve the condition. Patients are encouraged to participate in exercises that increases muscle strength as that can help protect the joints. Even the cardiovascular exercises such as walking, swimming, water exercises and low/non impact aerobic dance are now being recommended for those who can enjoy it. James Fries M.D., associate director of Stanford Arthritis Center says that "body systems including the joints, work better when they are used then when they are not used." (*Physician and Sports Medicine*, Jan. 1990, p.123). In the Resource section there is a listing of arthritis programs, articles and the address of the Arthritis Foundation where you can obtain more information.

Precautions

Don't do weight bearing asanas that jar the joints.

Recommendations

1. Do the poses in a slow, controlled static stretch .

2. Move through the fullest range of motion the joint is capable of.
3. Use the breath to help with the flow of energy and to increase circulation
4. Visualize the affected area moving easily with no pain or discomfort to assist the body to become stronger and healthier
5. Visualize your body in a perfect skeletal alignment with strong, flexible muscles holding your skeleton together in its perfect alignment
6. Try doing the standing yoga poses in a pool (water at 83 to 88 degrees F)
7. If you have rheumatoid arthritis wait until later in the day to practice as the morning stiffness will have abated.
8. If you have osteoarthritis practice earlier in the day before the wear and tear of the days activities have tired the affected joints.
9. If you are experiencing pain 2 hours after your yoga session then you need to scale down or modify your exercises.
10. It is very important to do the Preparation Poses you enjoy to warm up and also cool down.
11. Use the necktie to assist you in moving into the yoga asanas.
12. Light massage and heat or ice can help with pain as well as accupuncture.

Recommended Asanas for Arthritis

Preparation Poses: For Warm Up and Cool Down
    All presented in Unit 3 are suitable but if there is an area of your body that is bothered by them do the pose very gently or DON'T do at all if there is pain.

Asanas:
    Mountain Pose (figure 3.12 on page 18)
    Cobra (figure 3.13 on page 19): Modification - if palms can not go flat to the mat make fists instead.
    Cat (figure 3.20 on page 24): same modification as above
    Dog (figure 3.21 on page 25): same modification as above
    Head of the Cow (figure 3.18 on page 22): use

necktie if needed. This pose is in the Arthritis Foundation Videotape of their PACE program (People with Arthritis Can Exercise)
    Shoulder Stand (figure 3.22 on page 26-27): Which ever variation feels good
    Crocodile Routine (figure 5.5 on page 63) of Swami Dev Murti as it is wonderful for the spine and the laughter part is helpful with pain control.

Almost all of the asanas are suitable if YOU feel comfortable doing them. Some may be more difficult to do than others such as the following:

    Lunge (figure 3.29 on page 34)
    Plank (figure 3.30 on page 34)
    Spinal Twist (figure 3.33 on page 37)
    Full Locust (figure 3.35 on page 38)

VISUAL CONCERNS

Yoga is an ideal activity for those with vision problems. What is of basic importance here is that the verbal cues and directions should be very precise with nothing left to the imagination. I thank each one of the visually impaired students I have had in yoga as they *taught* me a lot about teaching the asanas to them. The environment in which yoga is taught is a safe one for a blind person. They can feel comfortable as there is less movement among the class members and many poses are done on the floor thus there is less risk of falling. The visualization cues can help with the body image, and awareness of how the body can move is also enhanced. The benefits from the breathing and the relaxation are the same as for those who are sighted.

Precautions

If the vision problem (such as glaucoma or retina damage) could be worsened by bringing blood to the head do NOT do the inverted poses of Dog, Headstand Hang, or Headstand and do Chest Expansion for 5-10 seconds only.

Recommendations

1. If the directions for doing the poses are not clear ask a teacher to help you.

2. Try using a small, wooden manniken that is jointed and can be placed in the asana by the teacher. The student can then feel with the hands the shape and with this " image" through touching can then do the pose themself.

Yoga Eye Exercises

The eyes are moved by muscles, and they too can benefit from exercise. Relaxing exercises of the eyes are included in the practice of yoga, acupuncture, and acupressure. The yoga eye exercises involve movement, while the acupressure approach is through massage. All of these exercises increase the circulation to the eye muscles and can help relieve eyestrain and that tired feeling we have from time spent at the computer or reading. Doing these exercises while wearing contacts or glasses is all right, but you may prefer to remove them.

Two types of eye exercises will be taught: the hatha yoga eye exercises and the Chinese eye exercises. Following are the basic directions. Seat yourself comfortably. You do not move the head; *only the eyes* will move. Keep breathing normally and allow the rest of your body to become fully relaxed. These exercises are simple to do and can be done at almost any time or place.

Tracking to the Right and Left

1. Gazing straight in front of you, find a spot to be your center focal point.
2. Slowly and smoothly move the eyes to the right as far as they can go; now move them to the left as far as they can go. Repeat
3. Blink your eyes, then close them to rest.

Tracking Up and Down

1. Gazing straight in front of you, find a spot to be your center focal point.
2. Slowly and smoothly move the eyes up as far as they will go. (You can probably see the fringe of your hair.) Now slowly and smoothly move them down (Now you can probably see the side of your nose.) Repeat
3. Blink your eyes, then close them and allow them to rest.

Clock Tracking

1. Gazing straight in front of you, find a spot to be your center focal point; this is where the imaginary hands of the clock are attached.
2. Now, slowly and smoothly move your eyes up to 12 o'clock, then slowly around to 1 and 2 o'clock. At 3, the eyes should be as far to the right as they can go. Then move on to 4 and 5. At 6 o'clock the eyes are looking down. Continue on to 7 and 8. At 9 o'clock the eyes are over to the far left. Move on to 10, 11, and finally 12 o'clock, at which time you are gazing up as far as your eyes can go. Now reverse the movement, moving the eyes to 11, 10, 9, etc.
3. Finish by closing your eyes. Place your palms over them and allow them a few minutes torest. As you did these exercises, did you notice a feeling of warmth around the eyes? Did they water? These are common responses because the eyes are probably not used to doing these exercises. Exercising the eyes will not necessarily correct any eye problems, but it is a way of strengthening the muscles and improving circulation. Once you try them you will find they are very refreshing and relaxing and should be done periodically when you are studying.

Chinese Eye Exercises

These exercises involve a massaging action which is stimulating and increases the circulation to the eyes. The sinuses may also respond. You will notice this by the urge to sniff or blow your nose. An art student from China taught these exercises to one of our yoga classes and told us that children from pre-school age through teenage years do them during their school day.

Chinese Eye Exercise Directions
(See Fig. 7.9 for placement of hands)

1. Place thumbs in the corner of the eye on the boney area. Find a slight depression and press and move the

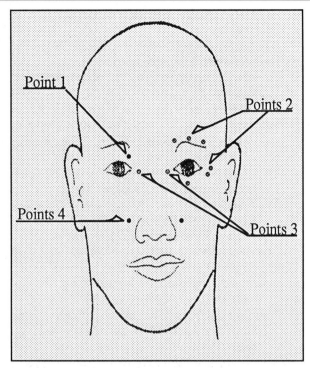

Figure 7.9. *Chinese Eye Exercises placement of hands*

thumbs in circles. Elbows are directed forward. Do 8 circular motions and them reverse direction and repeat.

2. The thumbs are on the temples. The index fingers are bent and massage across the bone on the eyebrow and below the eye opening of the skull. Do 8 wipes above and 8 below the eye.

3. Place the thumb and the finger on the bridge of the nose by the tear ducts and pull up pinching slightly 4 times. Do 4 more with the other hand.

4. Place the index fingers by the cheek bones in a depression near the nostrils of the nose and make 8 circular motions and reverse the direction for 8 more.

ADDICTIONS

There are many underlying causes for a persons tendency to become addicted to food, cigarettes, alcohol or illegal drugs. It is a complicated scene involving, genes, dysfunctional family units, lifestyle pressures such as stress, economic settings and lack of knowledge about the harmful effects of a substance that can lead one to an addicted state. Many people have been helped with their addiction when yoga was introduced to them. In the beginning it appears that a respect for the physical body is enhanced by doing the yoga asanas and pranayama. Thus a desire to take better care of the physical body develops. As a spin off the benefits from relaxation, imagery and music then come into play. Often people with an addiction are not comfortable with focusing on the inner self and will attempt to deny their feelings by escaping with the addiction. By being led through the gentle coping mechanisms taught in yoga, such as using the breath to calm oneself, an addicted person can better deal with a daily trauma or a crisis.

In 1973 in Tucson, Arizona the 3HO (Happy, Healthy and Holy Organization) a residential treatment program was developed. People coming here are alcoholics, cigarette smokers, recreational drug users, people with weight problems, relationship difficulties and stress problems. At the center they do hatha yoga, mantra-chanting, and pranayama. They also have opportunities for counseling, massage and eat vegetarian meals to assist with detoxifying and healing. People stay from one week to one month (or longer if necessary). A survey of the graduates between 1983 to 1986 indicated a recovery rate of 91%. This center is for those who want to change and are willing to work to make it happen. See the Resources section for additional information in articles and the address of 3HO.

There are no specific Precautions and Recommendations for addictions. All of the poses would be fine to do, with a lot of emphasis on the breath and relaxation.

WHEEL CHAIR YOGA

Yoga has been taught with success to those with multiple sclerosis, cerebral palsy, muscular dystrophy, Parkinsons disease and heart disease. The Hatha Yoga asanas can be modified to be done in wheel chairs. Using the neckties to assist with the body alignment is also helpful for those with a disability. Learning to use the breath to calm and to energize the body is also of great benefit for those who are handicapped in some way. The benefits of relaxation, music and visualization are the same for those with a disability or those who have none. In Ickwell Bury, England there is a residential center run by the Yoga for Health Foundation under the direction of Howard Kent. Here those with a disability can come and stay for any length of time and be supervised in doing yoga, learn pranayama, meditation, and enjoy eating nutritious meals. The staff consists of yoga teachers, a nurse, a physical therapist, massage therapist and a physician who makes calls and is available for consulting. Seminars and training programs in remedial yoga and medical problems are also sponsored by the center. You can find the address in the resources section.

For more information and for first hand accounts of yoga helping those with a disability you can refer to the books and articles listed in the resources section.

Recommendations

1. If possible do the yoga poses on a mat.
2. If staying in the chair lean away from the back so you are able to better use the muscles of your abdomen and back in the asanas to strengthen them.
3. Take the responsibility for your daily practice of yoga, and deep breathing.

Recommended Asanas for Those in Wheel Chairs

Neck Stretches (figure 3.1 on page 14)
Neck Turns (figure 3.2 on page 14)
Chest Expansion - with necktie (figure 3.19 on page 23)
Head of the Cow - with necktie (figure 3.18 on page 22)
Eye Exercises (figure 3.46 on page 46)
Lion (figure 3.31 on page 35)
Abdominal Lift (figure 3.27 on page 32)
Back Arch or a Cobra if on the mat (figure 3.13 on page 19)
Alternate Leg Stretch with necktie either in chair or on the mat (figure 3.11 on page 17)
Triangle - when done sitting it becomes a side bend (figure 3.25 on page 30)
Triangle Twist - when sitting place the opposite hand on the opposite leg or chair arm (figure 3.26 on page 31)
Shoulderstand - with the legs on the wall (figure 3.22b on page 26)
Fish pose - may need assistance to lift into arch (figure 3.23 on page 28)
Yoga sit back and if strong enough do the Yoga sit back AND UP (figure 3.32 on page 36)
Single and Both knees to chest (figure 3.5 and 3.16 on page 15, 20)
Fetus (figure 3.15 on page 20)
Feldenkrais kneeovers (figure 3.9 on page 16)
Try these routines:
   a. Moon Salute done in the chair.
   b. A sitting "Sun Salute" was developed and printed in the Yoga Journal. (see Resource Section)
   c. On the mat do the Crocodile Routine of Swami Dev Murti. (figure 5.5 on page 63)

SUMMARY

This unit shows ways that hatha yoga can be adapted to fit a persons individual needs. It is also emphasized that yoga is an activity recommended for older adults as well. So no matter your age, or special condition you can enjoy doing and benefit from yoga throughout your life.

RESOURCES

Menstrual Disorders
Iyengar B.K.S. *Light On Yoga.* New York, Shocken Books, 1966.
Iyengar, Geeta S., *Yoga: A Gem for Women:* New Delhi, Allied, 1983.
Fahri, Donna, "Yoga for Menstrual Cramps", *Yoga Journal,* May/June, 1986 p. 7-10.

Pregnancy
Arndt, Jennie. *Pre and Post Natal Yoga.* Video tape - $29.95. estimate 1-800-876-7798
Goldstein, Leslie. *Relax with Yoga During Pregnancy,* Nityanada Institute. Audio tape with foldout guide.
  $11.95 estimate. 1-800-876-7798
Jordan, Sandra. *Yoga for Pregnancy ,* St. Martins Press.
Music tapes for Infants and Children
LULLABY FOR THE HEARTS OF SPACE, Kevin Braheny 42b-6 Pyramid Books and New-Age Collection.
  35 Congress st. P.O. Box 48 Salem, MA 01970. $10.98 estimate.
LULLABY RIVER A04430. Red Rose Gallerie, P.O. Box 1859, Burlinggame, CA 94011
  1-800-451-LOVE $9.95 estimate.

Back Problems/ Neck Injury
Setterberg, Fred. "How I Got My Back Up", *In Health.* March/April 1990, p. 40-49.
Schatz, Mary Pullig, M.D. "Living With Your Lower Back", *Yoga Journal.* July/August 1984.

Scoliosis
Hatlett, Larry. "Hatha Yoga and Scoliosis",*Yoga Journal.* September/October 1982, p. 53-54.
Miller, Elise Browning. "Yoga for Scoliosis", *Yoga Journal.* May/June 1990, p. 66-75, 105-6.

Arthritis
Gach, Michael Reed. "Morning Stretches for Aching Joints," *Yoga Journal,* September/October 1989, p. 19-28.
Samples, Pat. "Exercise Encouraged for People With Arthritis" . *Physician and Sports Medicine.* Vol 18,
  No. 1 Janurary 1990, p.123-125, 127.
Arthritis Foundation, Box 19000, Atlanta, GA 30326.
Fries, James MD. and Kate Lorig. "The Arthritis Helpboook". Stanford CA. Arthritis Center.
International Yoga Centre, Highfield Lenham, Nr. Maidstone, Kent, Me172EX Telephone # Lenham 431
  (858431) Attn: Karen Honeybun or Peter Lovelock

Visual Concerns
Marantz-Henig, Robin and Judith Groch. "Too Close for Comfort. *American Health-Fitness of Body and
  Mind.* April 1985, p. 62-71.

Addictions
Lefton, Judith. "Yoga Therapy for Addictions" *Yoga Journal,* March/April 1990, p. 25-30.
Shepherd, Bliss. "Dealing with Our Addictions". *Yoga Journal,* November/December 1988, p. 49, 103.
3HO SuperHealth, 2545 N. Woodland Rd. Suite 600, Tucson, AZ 85749

Wheel Chair
Brosnan, Barbara. *Yoga for Handicapped People.* Souvenir Press, London, 1982.
Bell, Lorna and Eudora Seyfer. *Gentle Yoga.* Igram Press, Cedar Rapids, Iowa, 1982.
Hall, Rosemary. "Seated Sun Salutation." *Yoga Journal* March/April, 1986.

Older Adults
Birkel, Dee Ann and Susan Birkel Freitag. *Forever Fit: Step by Step Program of Physical Activity for Older
  Adults.* New York, Plenam Publishing, Insight Press, 1991-92.

General Sports Warm-up and Cool Down

Neck Turns (figure 3.2 on page 14)
Neck Stretches (figure 3.1 on page 14)
Body Rolls (figure 3.3 on page 14)
Wall Stretch (figure 3.6 on page 15)
Head of Cow (figure 3.18, 8.1 on page 22, 93)
Chest Expansion (fig. 3.19, 8.2 on page 23, 92)
Spinal Twist (figure 3.33, 8.3 on page 37, 93)
Dog (figure 3.21, 8.4 on page 25, 93)
Alternate Leg Stretch (fig. 3.11, 8.5 on page 17, 93)
Sitting Forward Bend (figure 3.17 on page 21)
Moon Salute Routine (figure 3.46 on page 46)
Sun Salute Routine (figure 3.47 on page 47)

YOGA AND SPORTS

*"Every athletic career, no matter how modest or lofty, is a journey.
On any journey, we need a clear map, a sound vehicle and sufficient quality of fuel.
The mind is the map, the body the vehicle and the emotions the fuel."*
...Dan Millman, *The Warrior Athlete. xiii*

Many champion athletes have enjoyed doing yoga - Jean Claude Killey the French Olympic Ski Champion; the golfers Jack Nicklaus and Gary Player; boxer Sugar Ray Robinson; tennis player John McEnroe; dancers Ruth St. Denis, Marge Champion, Shirley MacLaine and numerous others. Football teams such as the Washington Redskins and the Pittsburgh Steelers began doing yoga like stretches to prevent injuries. They have all noticed improvement in their flexibility and their range of motion. Learning more efficent use of the breath can also help with the energy level. The practice of relaxation in the corpse position also can have a carry over to being relaxed as you are executing a particular sports skill. A relaxed muscle moves more freely and easily. Being too tense can inhibit the flow of your movement.

Bud Winter, the track coach at San Jose State from 1940-1970, brought attention to the value of relaxation in sports. His track athletes earned thirty-seven world records. At one time his runners held all ten world records for sprinting and made an outstanding showing for the United States at the 1968 Olympics in Mexico City. He had taken the relaxation techniques that he had helped develop at the United States Naval Aviation School at Del Monte Pre-Flight center during World WarII and applied them to coaching his track athletes. In the early research with the Navy pilots they "found that in all sports and highly specialized skills, such as flying a plane, the greatest enemy to peak performance was hypertension - that is too much tension." (p.4 *Relax and Win,* Bud Winter) They also discovered you should relax the muscles that are not necessary to perform the task at hand. So he coached his atheletes to put out nine-tenths effort,

as going all out at 100% caused "tying up", wasting their energy and causing the muscles to perform less efficiently. His athletes were determined mentally but stayed loose and relaxed physically. In his book, *Relax and Win,* he applies his technique to boxing, baseball, skiing, swimming, basketball, bowling, golf, tennis, soccer, football and track and field. Being relaxed also can speed up the reaction time, which is a key element in executing many sports skills.

The mind's involvement in sports performance is getting more attention now as well. "Mental practice" is a form of imagery or visualization discussed in Unit 5. A whole new type of video tapes has been developed around this idea of viewing the worlds best performer who executes a skill flawlessly. Then you image yourself doing the same movement. When you combine this "image" with being in a relaxed state you can enhance your performance. Bud Winter advises having a "mental set" such as being "cool and confident." This can help you as you perform later. See Table 8.1 for examples of situations and slogans from Bud Winter's Mental Sets.

GENERAL SPORTS WARM-UP AND COOL-DOWN

Using the yoga poses as a warm up and cool down routine for athletic activity can help prevent injuries. The yoga poses are done without bouncing or force and are executed in a slow relaxing manner as you concentrate on what the body is feeling. This concentration leads to a greater awareness of the body's movement and can carry over to the execution of the sports skill.

Table 8.1.   *Bud Winter's Mental Sets*

Situation	Mental Set Slogan
Studying for an examination	*"I am going to be relaxed and learn."*
Running a race	*"I am going to run fast and loose."*
Asking for a date with a special person	*"I am going to be happy, interesting, poised, and thoughtful."*
Ringing doorbell on first date	*"I am going to do everything possible to make this person happy."*
In a crisis situation	*"Stay calm. I will beat this. Stay Calm."*
Giving a speech	*"I am going to be cool, poised, and humorous."*

Bud Winters, *Relax and Win-Champion Performance in Whatever You Do.,*p. 50-51

Table 8.2 is a list of yoga poses that would function as a General Warm-up and Cool-Down routine. In addition to these poses add those listed under the sport heading that is of special interest to you.

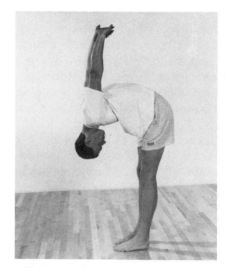

Figure 8.1.   *Chest Expansion*

Table 8.2.   *General Sports Warm-up and Cool Down*

Neck Turns (figure 3.2 on page 14)
Neck Stretches (figure 3.1 on page 14)
Body Rolls (figure 3.3 on page 14)
Wall Stretch (figure 3.6 on page 15)
Head of Cow (figure 3.18, 8.6 on page 22, 93)
Chest Expansion (figure 3.19, 8.1 on page 23, 92)
Spinal Twist (figure 3.33, 8.4 on page 37, 93)
Dog (figure 3.21, 8.7 on page 25, 93)
Alternate Leg Stretch (figure 3.11, 8.5 on page 17, 93)
Sitting Forward Bend (figure 3.17 on page 21)
Moon Salute Routine (figure 3.46 on page 46)
Sun Salute Routine (figure 3.47 on page 47)

Running/Walking

Toe Hold Leg Lift (figure 8.2)
Kneeovers (figure 3.9 on page 16)
Abdominal Lift (figure 3.27 on page 32)
Balance Posture (figure 3.41 on page 43)

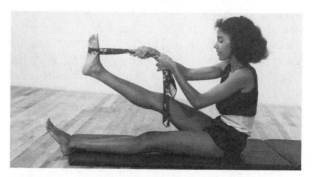

Figure 8.2.   *Toe Hold Leg Lift*

Racket Sports

Chest Expansion (figure 8.1)
Lunge (figure 3.29 on page 34)
Tree (figure 3.24 on page 29)
Balance Posture (figure 3.41 on page 43)
Kneeovers (figure 3.9 on page 16)

Volleyball

Back push up (figure 8.3)
Lunge (figure 3.29 on page 34)
Abdominal Lift (figure 3.27 on page 32)
Knee overs (figure 3.9 on page 16)
Cobra (figure 3.13 on page 19)

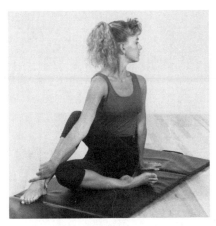

Figure 8.3. *Back Push-Up*

Golf

Spinal Twist (figure 8.4)
Balance Posture (figure 3.41 on page 43)
Tree (figure 3.24 on page 29)
Cobra (figure 3.13 on page 19)

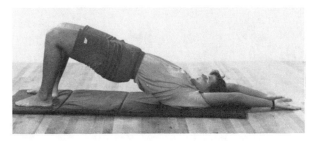

Figure 8.4. *Spinal Twist*

Weight Lifting

Alternate Leg Stretch (figure 8.5)
Toe Hold Leg Lift (figure 8.2)
Balance Posture (figure 3.41 on page 43)
Abdominal Lift (figure 3.27 on page 32)
Cobra (figure 3.13 on page 19)

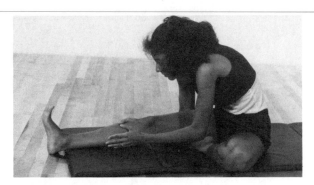

Figure 8.5. *Alternate Leg Stretch*

Basketball

Head of Cow (figure 8.6)
Dog (figure 8.7)
Lunge (figure 3.29 on page 34)
Abdominal Lift (figure 3.27 on page 32)
Knee Overs (figure 3.9 on page 16)
Cobra (figure 3.13 on page 19)

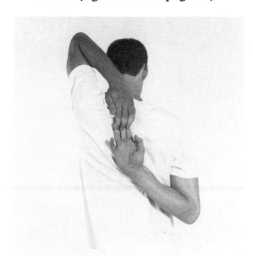

Figure 8.6. *Head of Cow*

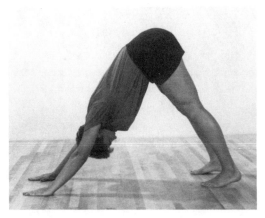

Figure 8.7. *Dog*

SUMMARY

In addition to the above Hatha Yoga routines it is fun to do the partner routine (see Unit 3) as it can add to the feeling of teamwork and camaraderie between the members of a team. It is also fun to do some massage activities at the end of a practice. (See Unit 9.) Also remember that many athletes value the use of a Flotation Tank (Unit 5) and its positive influence on their sports performance through mental practice and release of stress.

RESOURCES

Christensen, Alice. *The American Yoga Association Beginner's Manual.* New York, A Fireside Book, Simon & Schuster, Inc., 1987.

Couch, Jean and Weaver, Nell. *Runner's World Yoga Book.* Mountain View, Calif.: Runner's World Publications, Inc., 1979.

Folan, Lilias. *Lilias, Yoga, and Your Life.* New York, Macmillan Publishing Co., Inc., 1981.

Jackson, Ian Scott, *Yoga and the Athlete,* World Publications, Mountain View, CA. 1975.

Leonard, George. *Mastery.* Dutton/New American Library. 1990.

Millman, Dan. *The Way of the Peaceful Warrior.* Los Angeles, J.P. Tarcher Publisher, 1980.

_____ *The Warrior Athlete : Body, Mind and Spirit.* Walpole, New Hampshire, Stillpoint Publishing. 1979.

Winter, Bud. *Relax and Win : Championship Performance In Whatever You Do.* San Diego, CA. A.S. Barnes and Company, Inc. 1981.

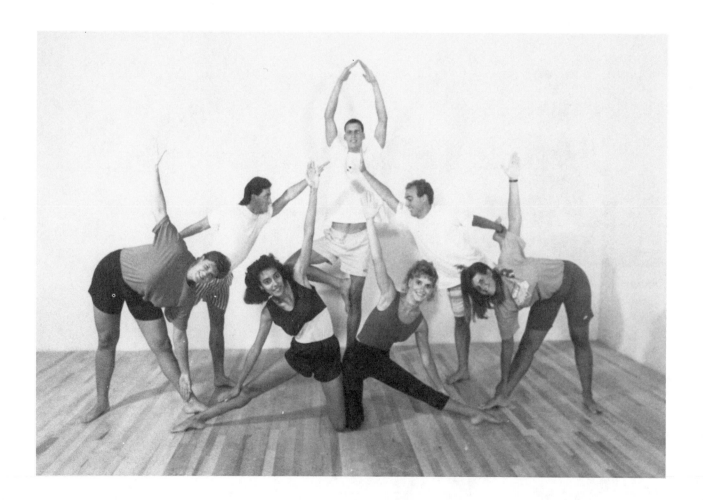

OTHER WAYS TO BODY AND MIND AWARENESS

*"If of thy mortal goods thou are bereft,
And from thy slender store two loaves alone to thee are left,
Sell one, and with the dole- Buy hyacinths to feed thy soul."*
. . . Mohammedan sheik (1183 -1206)

As your practice with yoga grows you become more aware of your whole self and how you function: your habits regarding your posture and how you move. This unit will present the basics about other approaches to body/mind integration and alignment. Some of these "body therapies" were developed by people who did yoga and meditation. Each approach will be briefly described and in the resource section under each heading there will be a listing of articles, books, audio tapes and the address of where to write for information and names of teachers or practioners who are trained and/or certified. I have personally experienced and enjoyed all of these approaches discussed in this unit.

soak for 30 minutes in a bath tub of hot water to which you have added one quart of apple cider vinegar (not the synthetic type). She recommends to all her clients to do this following their visit to her as this alleviates the muscle soreness that comes from increasing the circulation and affecting the position and alignment of the body parts worked on. Try this if you have over done in any form of exercising such as the first day back in an aerobics dance class or the first few days of athletic practice if you have been inactive for a while.

MASSAGE THERAPY

This technique is directed toward working with the muscles and joints of the body to relieve tension and improve alignment and circulation. Those trained in it have studied anatomy and physiology as well as a variety of massage techniques such as Swedish, Shiatsu, and reflexology. It is very helpful if you are recovering from an injury or have a chronic alignment problem caused by scoliosis, for example. The American Association of Massage Therapists maintains a list of those certified to practice.

It is becoming popular to use some massage techniques along with the counterposes in yoga classes to help alleviate muscle tension. (Fig. 9.1) A tip I learned from my massage therapist that also relieves muscle tension is to

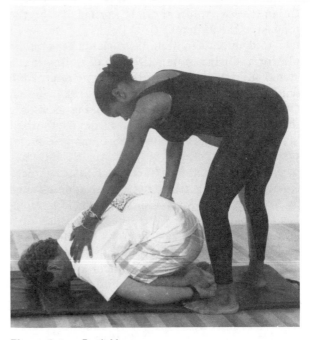

Figure 9.1. *Back Massage*

CHIROPRACTIC

"Look well to the spine for the cause of disease."
. . . Hippocrates, 4th Century B.C.   Greece.

The word "chiropractic" comes from a Greek word for manual medicine. Dexter Nardella, D.C. explains the practice of chiropractic as "a clinical science which is based upon: 1) the law of biology which states that there is a capacity in all living things to be well (Homeostasis); 2) the theory of physiology that the nervous system provides total control of the body's functions; 3) the chiropractic hypothesis that health in the nervous system relates to health in the body; and 4) the *major* premise of chiropractic - there is a relationship between the framework of the spine and the health of the nervous system.

The art of chiropractic lies in the use of the hands to detect minute changes in spinal function and to correct those changes using refined techniques of spinal adjustment or manipulation.

Chiropractic's success with a variety of diseases is well documented. And yet its purpose in caring for people is not to treat disease. The purpose of the chiropractor is to correct nerve interference from the spine (vertebral subluxation). You might say that chiropractors care for the well-being of the entire person who has the disease rather treating a specific disease only.

Chiropractic is now making a contribution to the Sports Medicine scene as it is now a component of the United States Olympic Committee's Medical Staff, primarily at the request of the athletes. Greg Louganis, winner of two gold medials in diving, struck his head on the platform during competition and following a spinal adjustment by a chiropractor he returned to win his third gold medal in the 1984 Seoul Olympics. Chiropractic is also being used as a therapy or treatment for athletes from the football teams of Miami Dolphins, San Francisco 49ers; the competitors at the 1987 Pan American Games in Indianapolis; the 1988 United States Greco-Roman Wrestling team; individual athletes such as Bruce Jenner, Suzy Chaffee, Francie Larrieu, Henry Rono, and Dwight Stone. The use of a chiropracter as a "team doctor" for elementary children to the olympic level athletes has been growing in popularity. 'Weekend athletes" can also benefit from a visit to a chiropractor.

ALEXANDER TECHNIQUE

This Technique was developed by F.M. Alexander, an actor from Australia, around 1900. He developed a problem with hoarsness of his voice which could not be explained by the medical community. In an attempt to find a cause he placed mirrors around his London flat to observe himself and eventually discovered that he threw his head back when speaking. This inhibited the flow of energy to his vocal chords and affected his speech. Out of this discovery he developed a system of observation by self and also by an Alexander teacher who would then help change the clients bad movement and alignment habits as observed in their daily activities.   Several prominent men of the day; playright George Bernard Shaw, author Aldous Huxley, educator John Dewey, were among those who learned and practiced the Alexander technique.

In this technique a person works with you giving you directions and gently touching you where you need a correction. A session lasts from 30-60 minutes. This technique is very popular with musicians and actors and is taught in many schools of music and theater around the world. The outcome is that a person becomes "educated" about how the performance of daily habits of movement can be changed to be done with less tension and increased lightness, fluidity and enhanced poise. Following in Fig. 9.2 two yoga students are gently working with the alignment of the neck and shoulders.

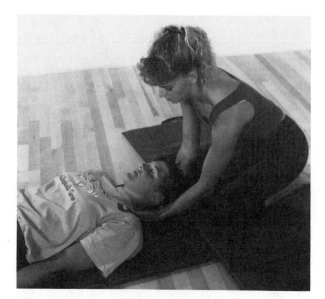

Figure 9.2.   *Alexander Technique*

FELDENKRAIS METHOD

This approach to body work was developed by Moshe Feldenkrais, Ph D., in the 1940's. Russian by birth, educated as a physicist, a mechanical and electrical engineer with a science doctorate from the Sorbonne, he became interested in the body's mechanics. He was an European champion in Judo holding a black belt and had spent time in India studying yoga. His growing interest in body movement expanded when an old soccer injury to his knee became a problem and he then began studying ways to help himself. Out of this study and interest evolved his two teaching methods; 1) "Functional Integration" (FI), which is hands on work practiced one to one and 2) "Awareness Through Movement" (ATM), which consists of simple movement exercises which are usually taught in a class. Reports of his work led to people going to Israel to be trained by him and to his becoming an author.

The basis for this body work is to use simple, non-habitual movement and to link this movement with the nervous system and the ways we learn. Developing a new movement pattern can stimulate the brain and break old harmful habits of movement and alignment. (See Fig. 9.3) His methods have been researched and are now taught by over 300 practioners worldwide. His program of movement has been taught to those with cerebral palsy, brain and spinal cord injuries as well as famous people such as "Dr. J." Julius Erving of basketball fame, violinist Yehudi Menuhin, anthropologist Margaret Mead and film director Peter Brook. He always emphasized that his technique did not "cure" but that if a person had trouble with movement he could probably improve the movement and thereby improve their health and wellbeing.

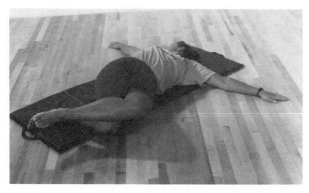

Figure 9.3a.   *Feldenkrais Legs*

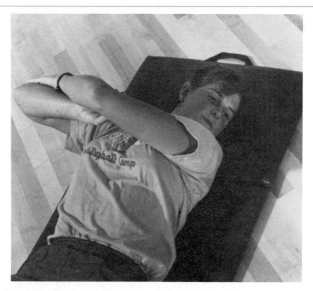

Figure 9.3b.   *Feldenkrais Arms*

TRAGER WORK

Milton Trager M.D., was born in Chicago and at sixteen moved to Miami where he was training as a boxer. He developed an interest in working with the body and helping people in his neighborhood and on Miami Beach with their aches and pains. In 1941 he received a Doctorate of Physical Medicine from the Los Angeles College of Drugless Physicians and during World War II he worked in the Physical Therapy Departmemt of the Navy. At the age of forty-one he tried to get admitted to American medical schools but all seventy that he applied to turned him down as they thought he was to old. He was accepted into Universitarie Autonoma de Guadalajara in Mexico where they organized a clinic for him to treat polio victims. He received his medical degree in 1955 and went to Hawaii. Here he met Maharishi Mahesh Yogi and became interested in Transcendental Meditation. People heard of his body work and many of those he had helped encouraged him to teach his method to others. Finally in 1977 he closed his private medical practice in Honolulu and the Trager Institute located in Mill Valley, California was founded. There are now well over 2000 students throughout the world and more than 300 practitioners. To locate one see the resource section for the address.

The Trager method like the Feldenkrais has two basic approaches: 1)The practioner works with the client on a massage table. This is called

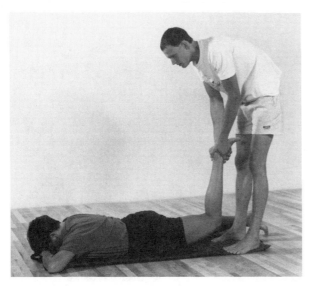

Figure 9.4.   *Tragering*

"Trager Psychophysical Integration "(TPI), and consists of gentle rolling, rocking, and wavelike motions -- a sort of subtle dance between practitioner and client. (See FIG. 9.4) The practioner begins the session by getting into a state of "hook up" which is used to connect with the client in a gentle "meditation in motion" style. The experience of TPI is very relaxing as the touch is very light and feathery and never forceful. The goal is to help allow the mind to help the body to release the tension - not increase the tension by attacking it and causing discomfort. 2) This approach is known as "Mentastics", a word coined by Dr. Trager from "mental gymnastics." This is done in a class with a teacher leading you through some shaking, loosening types of exercise. You are using the motion in the tissue, muscles and joints to produce a sensory feeling that will enter the central nervous system and allow the mind to connect to the muscles forming new sensory-motor patterns. The result is that the body will feel lighter and then will stand and move lighter resulting in a new ease in how daily activities are performed.

The Trager Method has been of help to many afflicted with polio, muscular dystrophy, multiple sclerosis as well as those with old injuries and body alignment problems. For already healthy people, Trager work has a profound lightening and loosening effect on both body and mind.

ACUPUNCTURE AND ACUPRESSURE

Acupuncture and acupressure, two ancient Chinese forms of healing are based on the principle of balance and harmony. There is a life-force energy running through our bodies which the Chinese call chi or ki, (called prana in yoga, see Unit 4). This energy should run freely along pathways of energy called meridians. Along these meridians are sites, the acupuncture and acupressure points, where needles are inserted or pressure applied to help the energy run smoothly. If there is an imbalance of energy then a person will experience symptoms of disease.

The diagnosis of a patient is very specific and based on asking many questions, looking and listening. Chinese medicine is very closely tied to nature and it is often believed that imbalances of the body arise from overexposure to cold, hot, damp or wind.

There are two aspects of chi, and these are yin and yang. The two energies have opposing qualities that must be in balance and work together for the body to be healthy. The table 9.1 below shows qualities of yin and yang.

You can use pressure or acupuncture sites to help restore the balance of energy in the body. In the following diagrams are some points you can use to help yourself, or have someone else use for you. Remember that it is important to use fairly strong, evenly applied pressure on both sides of the body for a bilateral point, and to press for 2-3 minutes, then move to another site, or wait a few minutes and repeat the pressure.

Table 9.1.

YIN	YANG
Feminine	Masculine
Night	Day
Lower	Upper
Back	Front
Soft	Hard
Contracting	Expanding
Negative	Positive
Deficiency	Excess
Cold	Hot

Instructions for Locating Sites

1. Concentration, Memory point: Located on a line straight up from the nose, over the top of the head in a hollow just behind the crown.

2. Nasal congestion point: Run finger up the side of the nose until it reaches the top of a triangle of cartilage.

3. Toothache point: Located in the corner of the jaw and found by running finger up towards ear (approximately 1 inch) until it falls in hollow.

4. Cough and asthma points : 2 points- Located just over and behind the bone in the hollow of the throat. 2nd point on midline of the body even with the level of the nipples.

5. Stomach ache point: Located on the midline of the front of the body halfway between the bottom of the sternum and the navel.

6. Water retention and menstrual pain/ problems: Located on the line going down the leg from the medial side of the kneecap, approximately 5 fingers distance from the kneecap and over the round top of the bone.

7. Water retention and menstrual pain/ problems: Located up from the inside of the ankle bone 4 fingers distance and back from the shinbone approximately 1/2 to 3/4 inch.

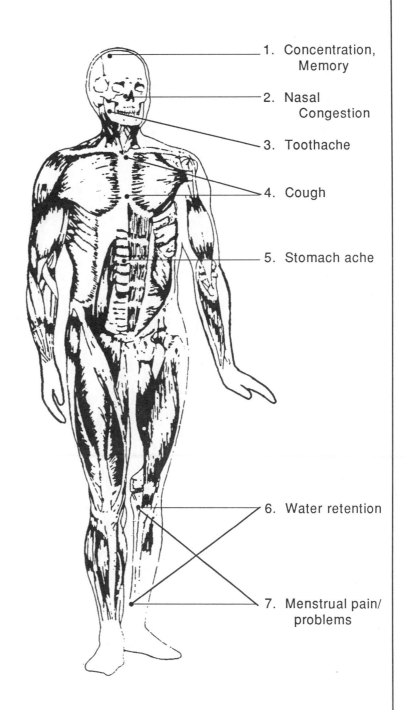

1. Concentration, Memory
2. Nasal Congestion
3. Toothache
4. Cough
5. Stomach ache
6. Water retention
7. Menstrual pain/ problems

Instructions for Locating Sites

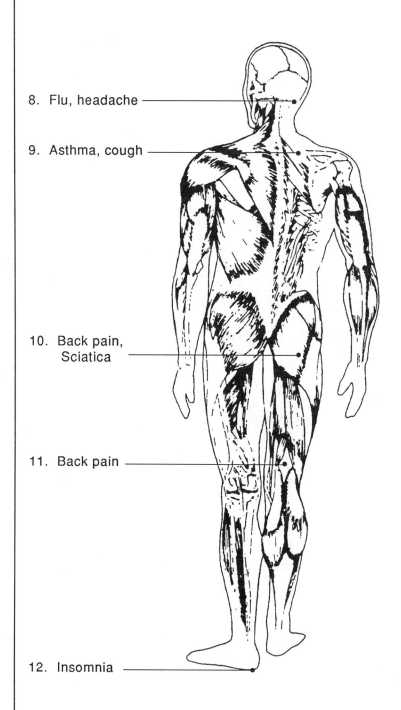

8. Flu, headache

9. Asthma, cough

10. Back pain, Sciatica

11. Back pain

12. Insomnia

8. Flu and Headache point: Located in a hollow where the skull meets the neck muscles on the back of the head. This point will be very sore if you are coming down with the flu or a cold.

9. Asthma and cough points (3 points each side): Located approximately 1 inch, 1 1/2 inch and 2 inches out from the 1st thoracic vertebrae which is at the level of the shoulders.

10. Back pain and sciatica point: Located just lateral to the center of each buttock. You will be able to tell when you have located this point because it gives a strong reaction.

11. Back pain point: Located on the crease in the center of the back of the knee and is easiest to find and apply pressure to while the knee is bent.

12. Insomnia point: In the center of the heel on the bottom of the foot.

Instructions for Locating Sites

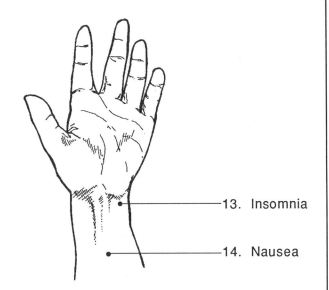

13. Insomnia point: Located just over the bone on crease of the wrist on a line running straight up the arm from the little finger.

14. Nausea, morning and carsickness point: Located on the inside of the wrist between the middle tendons and up the distance found by placing 4 fingers close together on the wrist crease.

15. Nosebleed point: Located on the outside corner of thumbnail. It is most effective to hold a burning stick of incense near the site to stop bleeding.

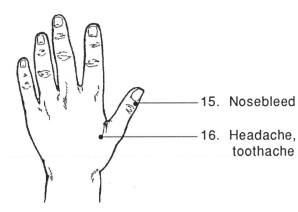

16. Headache and toothache point: Located at the top of the fleshy mound found by bringing thumb next to hand. Press down on the top of the crease nearest wrist, and inward towards the fingers, while index finger is pressing up from the bottom. This gives a strong reaction.

17. Hiccups point: Located on the ear where the top part curves in and flattens out.

18. Headache, hangover point: Located on the ear lobe.

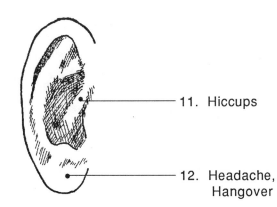

13. Insomnia
14. Nausea
15. Nosebleed
16. Headache, toothache
11. Hiccups
12. Headache, Hangover

Drawings by Lydia Gerbig, a Ball State University graduate.

TAI CHI CHUAN

Tai Chi Chuan is almost as old as yoga and it is also based on the theory of life force which in Chinese is referred to as "Chi". Tai Chi is a series of poses that are connected into routines of varrying lengths. Popular here in the United States is the 24 Step routine. The theory of Yin and Yang, discussed in the acupuncture section, is a concept that is also present in the practice of Tai Chi.

Tai Chi is done in a slow manner with a very controlled, smooth style that looks effortless but is not as the body is controlled and moved with energy and awareness. The use of the breath and balance are important components as well. It can improve posture, flexibility, muscular strength, balance, breath control, concentration and also lower stress. Once Tai Chi is learned it can be practiced for the rest of ones life with no expense just as yoga can be done.

SUMMARY

If you are enjoying your Hatha Yoga and like this approach to exercise you will probably enjoy doing any of the above programs also. These are all approaches that can be enjoyed throughout a person's life.

I would like to end this book by sharing the meaning of the Indian Greeting "Namaste" with you as it is interpreted by Ram Dass in his book *Grist for the Mill*, Unity Press.

Namaste

"In India when we meet and part we often say, '*NAMASTE,*' which means
I honor the place in you where the entire universe resides,
I honor the place in you of love, of light, of peace.
I honor the place within you where if you are in that place in you and I am in that place in me, there is
  only one of us."

RESOURCES

Thompson, Keith. "The Future of The Body", *Yoga Journal,* May/June 1989. p.38-45,97.

Massage
James Bowling, Executive Secretary/Treasurer, American Massage and Therapy Association, P.O. Box 1270, 310
    Cherokee St., Kingsport, TN 37660. Phone (615) 245-8071.
Downing, G., *The Massage Book,* New York 1972, Random House.
Inkeles, G., *The New Massage,* New York 1980, Putnam.
Montagu, Ashley, *Touching,* New York 1978, Harper & Row

Chiropractic
Haldeman, S. "Spinal Manipulative Therapy in Sports Medicine."*Clinics in Sports Medicine ,* 1986, p. 277.

Alexander Technique
Alexander, F. Matthias.*Man's Supreme Inheritance.* London, Chaterson, 1946.
    _____ *The Use of the Self.* London, Re-Educational Publications, 1955.
    _____*Alexander Technique,* London, Thames and Hudson, 1974.

Barker, Sarah. *The Alexander Technique,* New York, Bantam, 1978.
Barlow, Wilfred. *The Alexander Principle,* New York, Random House, 1973.
American Center for Alexander Technique, Abraham Goodman House. 1 W. 67th St. New York NY (212) 799-0468.
The Society of Teachers of The Alexander Technique. 3b Albert Court, Kensington Gore, London SW 7, England. Telephone 01-589-3834.

Feldenkrais
Feldenkrais, Moshe. *Awareness Through Movement.* New York, Harper & Row, 1977.
_____ *The Elusive Obvious.* Cypertino, CA, Meta Publications, 1981.
Houston, Jean. *The Possible Human,* Los Angeles ,J. P. Tarcher, Inc., 1982.
Master, Robert and Jean Houston. *Listening to the Body.* New York, Delacorte Press, 1981.
Holmes, B.:" Moving Well with Feldenkrais". *Yoga Journal,* Janurary/February, 1984, pp. 30-32.
Rosenfeld, A: " Teaching the Body How to Program the Brain is Moshe's Miracle". *Smithsonian,* January 1981

Audio Tapes
Feldenkrais Guild. P.O. Box 11145, San Francisco, CA 94101
Grotte, Josef Della Ph.D. P. O Box 612, Westminster MA 01473.
Holmes, Bruce. 801 Madison Ave. Dept. J11. Evanston, IL 60202 (312) 869-3434.

Trager Method
Cavanaugh Carol, "The Work of Milton Trager," *The Yoga Journal,* Sept- Oct. 1982, p. 20-25.
Drury Nevill, *The Bodywork Book,* Prism alpha, P.O Box 778, San Leandro, CA 94577. 1984.
Trager Institute, 300 Poplar Avenue, Suite #5 Mill Valley, CA 94941.
Trager, Milton, M.D.

Acupuncture
Traditional Acupuncture Foundation, American City Building, Columbia, MD 21044.
Acupuncture Research Institute, 313 W. Andrix St., Monterey Park, CA 91754
Brady, Sally R. "Acupuncture and Me", *Good Housekeeping,* August 1987, p. 58, 60-62.
Rodarmor, William. "Acupuncture Comes of Age in America", *Yoga Journal,* March/April 1986, p. 26-29, 64.
Stein, Douglas. "Interview with Ji-Sheng Han", *Omni Magazine,* Feb. 1988, p. 81-2, 84-5,102-3.
Wagner, Lindsay and Robert M. Klein. "The Acupressure Face-Lift", *New Age Journal,*March/April, 1989 p. 29-34.
Wilson, Beth. "Acupuncture: Healing More Than Pain", *Changing Woman,* Summer 1988, p. 17-18.

Tai Chi Chuan
Directory of Teachers- Tai Chi Association, P.O. Box 56113, Atlanta GA 30343.
Dunn Terrence. "The Practice and Spirit of Tai Chi Chuan". *Yoga Journal,* Nov./Dec/ 1987.
Friedman, Milton. "Chungliang Al Juang- A Master of Moving Meditation." *New Realities,* May/June 1989. p. 11-20.
Miller, Don and Julian, "An Ancient Art Can Change Your Running". *Runner's World,* March 1982, p. 58-61, 89-90.
Perry, Paul. "Grasp The Bird's Tail", *American Health,* Jan/Feb. 1986, p. 58-63.
Evehock, Goh and Sieapany,Chia. *Ten Minutes to Health.* Reno, Nevada. CRCS Publications

APPENDICES

A.   **SKELETON FRONT VIEW**

      SKELETON BACK VIEW

B.   **MUSCLES FRONT VIEW**

      MUSCLES BACK VIEW

A APPENDIX

Skeleton Front View

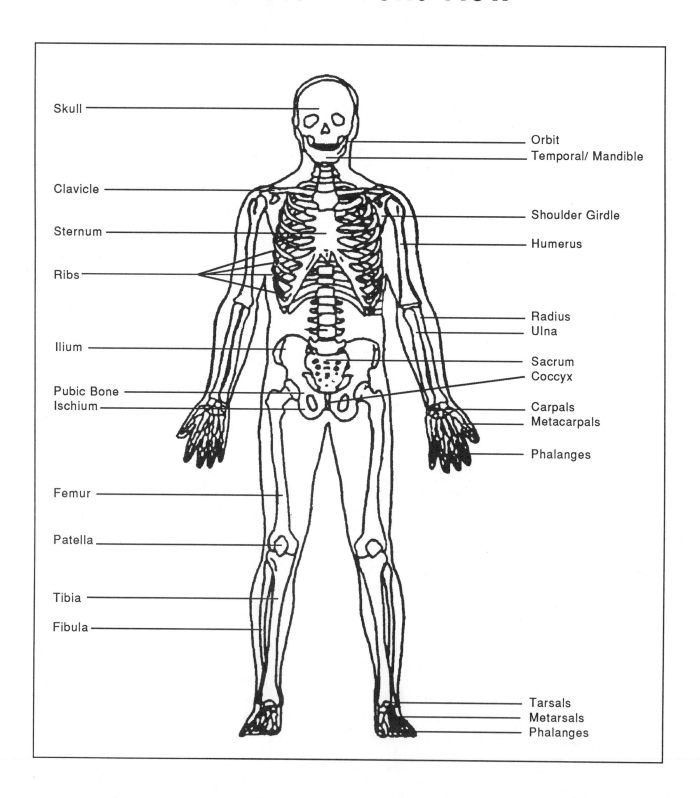

Skull

Clavicle

Sternum

Ribs

Ilium

Pubic Bone
Ischium

Femur

Patella

Tibia

Fibula

Orbit
Temporal/ Mandible

Shoulder Girdle

Humerus

Radius
Ulna

Sacrum
Coccyx

Carpals
Metacarpals

Phalanges

Tarsals
Metarsals
Phalanges

Skeleton Back View

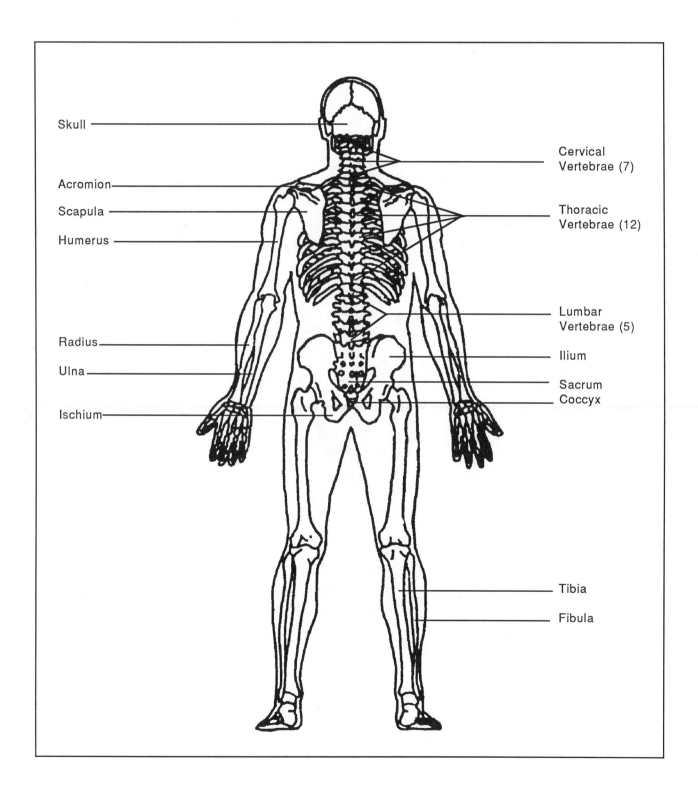

Skull

Acromion

Scapula

Humerus

Radius

Ulna

Ischium

Cervical
Vertebrae (7)

Thoracic
Vertebrae (12)

Lumbar
Vertebrae (5)

Ilium

Sacrum
Coccyx

Tibia

Fibula

B APPENDIX

Muscles Front View

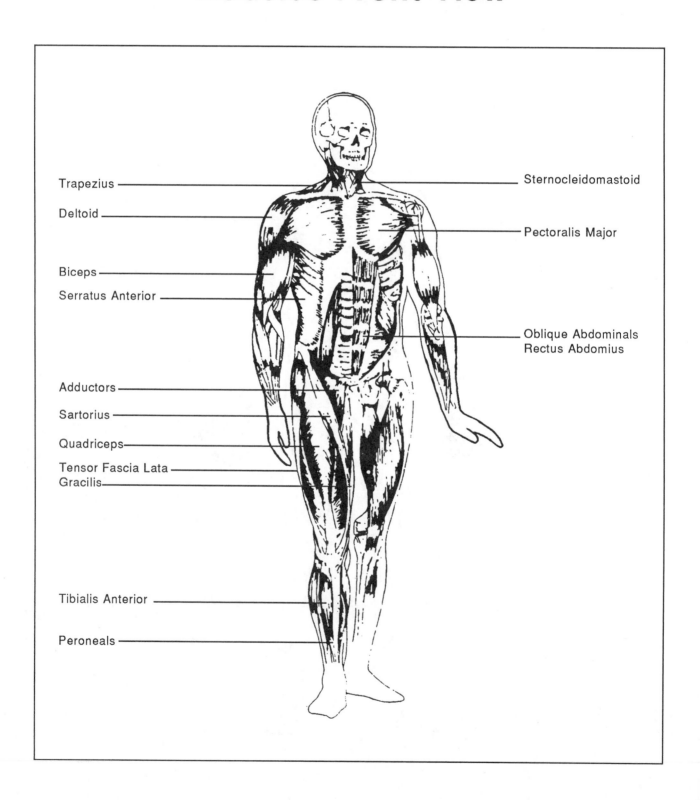

Trapezius

Deltoid

Biceps

Serratus Anterior

Adductors

Sartorius

Quadriceps

Tensor Fascia Lata

Gracilis

Tibialis Anterior

Peroneals

Sternocleidomastoid

Pectoralis Major

Oblique Abdominals
Rectus Abdomius

Muscles Back View

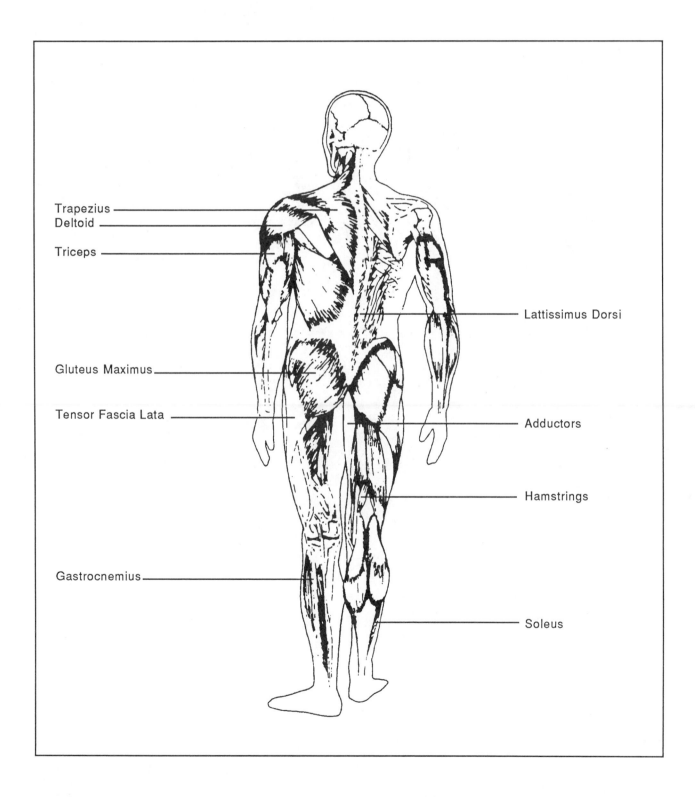

Trapezius

Deltoid

Triceps

Lattissimus Dorsi

Gluteus Maximus

Tensor Fascia Lata

Adductors

Hamstrings

Gastrocnemius

Soleus

INDEX